Sensitivity *is your*
SUPERPOWER

ISBN: 978-1-945446-88-7

Sensitivity *is your* SUPERPOWER

How to Harness Your Gifts, Fulfill Your
Purpose, and Create a Life of Joy

Karen Kan, MD

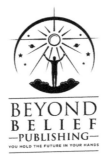

BEYOND
BELIEF
—PUBLISHING—
YOU HOLD THE FUTURE IN YOUR HANDS

This book is dedicated to all the Sensitive Souls
who bring light and love to our world.

Praise for
Sensitivity Is Your Superpower

"Dr Karen Kan has written the ONLY manual for an Empath or a Sensitive Soul. This is definitely on my students' MUST-read list."
– Richard Flook, Hay House Author of *Why Am I Sick?* and *How Can I Heal?*

"Every empath needs to read this book! Empaths are sensitive and gifted, not crazy and in need of *fixing!* Finally, an empathic medical doctor who talks the talk and walks the walk."
– Kate Moriah, Master Empath, Professional Psychic Medium, and Founder of Booming Eye Healing Arts

"Dr. Kan is a national treasure who shows the more sensitive souls among us how to not only function normally in modern society, but how to thrive and excel. She gives us remedies for many difficult situations, and creative ways to become super-powerful based upon hidden human abilities we are never taught about in school. I highly recommend this book, which illuminates a path less traveled, so more of us can recognize the benefits of taking this route."
– Ruth Rendely, Seraphim Blueprint Founder

"I've come across many healers over the years and Dr. Karen's programs are the only ones I invest in. She's *that* good. Her work is profound and you should definitely read this book if you want to raise your vibration!"
– Jeffrey Gignac, World-Renowned expert in Brainwave Stimulation and Entrainment, and founder of Passive Brain Fitness

"Sensitivity is Your Superpower is a book whose time has come! The world desperately needs us to step into the biggest version of ourselves.

To evolve our human spirit by connecting to more of ourselves. This book will empower you to be just that! Dr. Karen is such an inspirational and wise author, teacher and sage - *just Brilliant!*"

– Marcus Bird, Wellness Futurist, Founder of the Wellness Leadership Academy

"If ever there was an instruction manual on how to turn your sensitivity and empathy into Superpowers, *this is it!* This book is a game-changer!"

– Janna Arsenault, Founder of the Pain Freedom Method™

"This is a book that the world has been waiting for! Not only is Dr. Karen compassionate and comprehensive in her understanding of highly sensitive people, she shows us how to take what was once a problem and turn it into a Superpower. I absolutely love this book and I am recommending it to all of my clients!"

– Kimberley Banfield, Founder of Soulcology™

"As a Divine Channel and mentor, I help spiritually evolving women connect with their Divinity and embrace their power. Dr. Karen's book teaches Weather Magic, Transformational Telepathy™, Healing by Proxy-Prop™, and a whole host of other incredible, but easy-to-learn skills. If you have been looking for answers about your high sensitivity, you will be served. You will have clarity and knowledge to apply right away in your life, bringing your evolution to the next level and tapping into your infinite wisdom. It's a gift for you and for humanity!"

– Nicole Thibodeau, Oracle of Divine Transmissions, and #1 Bestselling Author of Evolutionary Healer

"As a highly sensitive person and a parent of a highly sensitive child, I am so grateful to learn that sensitivity is really a gift. It's our superpower! Dr. Karen's work has helped me and my family so much in learning how to channel and utilize this gift. This book is a must-read for any parent with a sensitive child."

– Rosie Sarandeva

"Of all the truly stellar tools that Creator has channeled through Dr. Karen, her new book, *Sensitivity is Your Superpower*, resides within a new *octave* of empowered support. This book might as well have wings. Thank you, Dr. Karen."

– Oliver LaPoint, Manager of Communications and Web Development

"As a parent of two little girls, I am thrilled to teach them what I'm learning in this book. I believe teaching children how to be calm in the face of adversity, and then showing them how their imagination can create a beautiful new reality, is one of the greatest things a parent can do. This book gets 5 stars!"

– Dr. Erin Kinney, Stress Reset Expert

"Dr. Karen has been a caring and compassionate mentor to me since I was 17. This may seem like a spiritual book to most people, but it is full of real-world practical ways to transform your life. I look at the success I've found in recent years, and can trace much of the foundation back to principles I've learned from Dr. Karen. Not only did she resolve my depression and bipolarity, but taught me how to use my sensitivities as my cardinal guides. Now that I've harnessed them, they are the wise sages in my ear, lighting the pathway in front of me. Get it - you won't regret it!"

– Jake Kent, Founder of Dilly Media

"I empower empaths to evolve out of energy bully abuse and remove relationship residue that is blocking their radiant relationship with themselves and others. Dr. Karen Kan has created a manual to show empaths and other sensitive souls how powerful they really are! Then provides tools to harness those superpowers. I highly recommend this book! It's a "must-have" for the bookshelf or digital reader of every sensitive soul!"

– Gwen Lepard, Luminary, Baggage Begone™ Facilitator, Leader of the Radiant Relationship Revolution, and #1 Bestselling Author of Evolutionary Healer

"This book radiates *Light*, *Love* and *Truth*; a true expression of Divinity. Eloquently written from an unbiased medical doctor's perspective. Your sensitivity can definitely be your superpower. Once you read it, you will be forever changed! Thank you Dr. Karen for showing us the way to experiencing our Divine gifts."

– Jenny Ngo, Intuitive Business Coach, Master Healer, and Founder of Purpose to Profits Coaching

"I struggled for years feeling symptomatic and isolated, not having anyone in the medical or energy community understand me. That's because I am a Sensitive Soul with ALL the symptoms on Dr. Karen's list, and needed guidance with dimensional imbalances and soul purpose. Every Sensitive Soul needs to stop struggling and start thriving. The first step is to read this book!"

– Lorena Calin, RN, BSN, Energy Healing Practitioner

"Thanks to Dr. Karen, I learned STOIM and Divine Muscle Testing™ and can now do "guru-level" self-healing! Not only do I no longer feel sick, weak and itchy all the time, I'm now physically stronger, happier, very self-sufficient, and much less emotional. And my income has tripled! I highly recommend this book to anyone who is highly sensitive and wants to harness their Superpowers! "

– Marion Mehrer, Executive Recruiter

"This book is an amazing gift! I feel that STOIM and TOLPAKAN™ Healing are the missing pieces in the healing journey for so many, including myself. I absolutely LOVE my work!"

– Josefin Kumlin, TOLPAKAN™ Healing Certified Practitioner and Founder of LifeFullness

"If every parent and child learned even a fraction of what's in this incredible book, I believe that we would all see less anxiety, depression and overwhelm. Why medicate your sensitive children when you can teach them how to harness their Superpowers instead?"

– Leslie Wendland, Co-Founder of the Sweaty Successful Moms

"What I've learned from Dr. Karen has been profound and life-changing. I have been able to overcome severe health challenges and do things I never thought I'd be able to do again! This book is so full of immense wisdom and light - you're going to love it!"

– Peggy Jo Wilhelm, TOLPAKAN™
Healing Certified Practitioner and
Graduate of the Light Warrior Training Camp™

"Kapow, kapow, kapow! This book delivers a punch! If you've ever wondered what is WRONG with you, Dr. Karen Kan has the answer: you've simply never been introduced to your sensitivity superpowers. Dr. Karen teaches you to stop hiding in the shadows and to emerge as the Sensitivity-Superhero that you truly are! It's a must-read!"

– Dr. Anna-Marie Wysynski, Medical Director of
Dr. Wysynski Bespoke Functional Medicine,
Menopausitive™ Facebook Group and
the Menopause 911™ Program

"I use Transformational Telepathy™ in my business with co-workers and clients and it really works! Dr. Karen has been an amazing mentor. This book is truly a Godsend to Sensitive Souls like me."

– Anna Rissberger, Founder of
whollybanAnna | the whollyogi

"Who doesn't want Superpowers? Whether you wish to learn how to influence the weather, send healing to a distant loved-one, or resolve conflict through telepathy, this book is fun and amazing!!"

– Mary Perry, Spiritual Healer, Seraphim Blueprint Teacher,
and Founder of Wings Unfurled

"Thanks to Dr. Karen, I've learned Divine Muscle Testing™ and do a lot of energy healing on myself and my family. I am so happy to recommend this book to my family and friends!"

– Sarah Campbell, Spanish Teacher

"Intuition, consciousness and healing with light and frequency...has gone from the depths of obscurity to becoming almost mainstream. This book comes at the perfect time to help us strip away what no longer serves us and *embrace* what does, so we can embody and experience our greatest dreams."

– Ayse Hogan, Founder and Chief of the International Academy of Universal Self-Mastery

"I traveled from Finland to New York to participate in Dr. Karen`s Light Warrior Training Camp. The experience was excellent and I decided to continue with TOLPAKAN™ Healing Method Level 1 and 2 Training. This year has included *major* ascensions in my life and the process continues with high expectations. I'll remember this evolution with gratitude and admiration."

– Matti Heinakari, MSc.(Eng), TOLPAKAN™ Healing Method Certified Practitioner, and Graduate of the Light Warrior Training Camp™

"Dr. Karen is an amazing healer, innovator, and teacher. She deeply cares about the truth and teaches people to heal themselves. This book is Divinely-inspired and I highly recommend it to anyone seeking to know their true Divine Self!"

– Lottie Cooper, Master Healer & Coach, Founder of Inspirational Counseling

"I've known Dr. Karen for a very long time, and she has guided and supported me in taking Quantum Jumps along my journey! If you know somehow that "you are more" - dive into her book and dare to believe. This book is Dr. K's perfect prescription for assistance with your life, your mission, and your ascension!"

– Cathy Hohmeyer, Quantum Chef, and Creator of the Nourishing Your Multidimensional Body program.

"You will be amazed by what you read in this book. I think every man, woman, and child can benefit from learning about their natural Superpowers, and Dr. Karen makes it easy and accessible!"

– Leanne Sheardown, Change Agent and founder of Happy Heads.

"It's absolutely amazing to read what my medical colleague, Dr. Karen Kan, has put together in this Superpower *manual*! Eye-opening and inspiring to say the least! I highly recommend it."

– Dr. Ailina Ismail, Fatigue Decoder Expert

"Everyone can learn how to thrive using the wisdom from this book, even if you don't think you're a Sensitive Soul. I highly recommend it!"

– Lisa Warner, Author of *The Simplicity of Self-Healing*

"Dr.Karen Kan is captivating! This book is packed with empowering novel possibilities. My close friends call me Superman - now I can harness my inner superpowers some more! I'm absolutely recommending it to my friends!"

– Anthony Frank Tan Wellness Entrepreneur

"Dr. Karen never ceases to amaze me. This book is beyond belief, yet when I look at all the incredible success Dr. Karen has had, and all the people she has helped, it makes perfect sense! Now I understand the secret to her success."

– James Loreto, Direct Sales Business Entrepreneur

"I'm thrilled this book is finally out! I feel like she saved my life. I trust Dr. Karen and you can too."

– Jessica Eckardt, Certified Dental Assistant

"The moment I listened to Dr. Karen on a telesummit, I knew I had to learn from her. I love her work and am 100% behind her mission. *This book may be one of the most important books to be published in this century so far!*"

– Natasha Lesiak, Administrative Assistant and Mother of Three

"Dr. Karen's *Superpower* book is SO fun and life-changing! Learning STOIM has shown me how to trust my inner guidance. Confidence uplifted!"

– Lianne Hofer, Founder of The Clutter Consultant

"I am a Chronic Health Specialist, and Health and Energy Coach, with over 23 years full time experience helping clients heal serious health conditions. So many people are suffering from chronic health conditions and in this book, Dr. Karen Kan offers up amazing wisdom as to why Sensitive people are so symptomatic. Then she guides the reader, step-by-step, on a unique journey to tap into their Superpowers! This book is incredible. "

– Lidia Kuleshnyk, Creator of the Apona Healing Method, www.AponaHealingMethod.com

"Normal is highly overrated. Thank you, Dr. Karen, for sharing your immense wisdom, insight, and inspiration on how we can all create and experience extraordinary lives!"

– Denise Peterson, Intentional Life Change Expert™

Contents

Acknowledgments

I used to think that I had to do everything and to figure out everything myself. Now I realize that the healthiest, wealthiest, and happiest people I know all have a team behind them, including mentors, coaches, assistants, friends, partners, tribe, and family members. I would like to share my deep gratitude for all the people who made the birth of this book possible.

Thank you, Keith Leon S., Maura Leon S., Karen Burton, Heather Taylor, Autumn Carlton, and the fantastic team at Beyond Belief Publishing for your patience and compassion. You made the publishing process a delight and I learned so much in the process!

Thank you to all my coaches and mentors—past, present, and future—who have believed in me, inspired me, and supported me, through thick and thin.

Thank you, Pat Jones, my first healer and spiritual teacher: for helping me connect to my spiritual gifts and for teaching me that it is my state of *being* that helps people more than my *doing*.

Thank you, Laura Day, my intuition teacher: you helped me believe in my natural intuitive gifts and your work helped me manifest my dream partner, James.

Thank you, Keith Leon S., my first coach: you gave me the courage to write and publish multiple books, and you helped me feel safe and loved when I was insecure about my future.

Thank you, T. Harv Eker: your amazing training programs helped me rewire my consciousness from scarcity to abundance and made me the confident speaker and trainer I am today.

Thank you, Jim Kaspari: you convinced me to hire my first assistant (I resisted, big time) and proved to me that taking risks and trusting the Universe brings in more money.

Thank you, Margaret Lynch Raniere: you introduced me to Rhys Thomas' Life Purpose Profiles and helped me heal the unsupportive energy patterns in my chakras that were blocking my success.

Thank you, Dr. Bradley Nelson: your amazing training programs, The Emotion Code and The Body Code, helped me release my Heart Wall, heal my ancestry, and step into my role as an entity-healing expert.

Thank you, Dr. Frank Kinslow: your Quantum Entrainment technique helped me experience *Eufeeling*, and I finally stopped feeling guilty for not meditating the "normal" way. You've radically changed my life for the better!

Thank you, Tamara Joy Patterson: you shifted my consciousness around entities from fear to love. Thank you for being my trusted guide when I had off-the-wall entity questions and had no one else to turn to.

Thank you, Jenny Ngo: you encouraged me to be a speaker on the "From Heartache to Joy Global Telesummit." Because of you, my work is now impacting thousands. Thank you for being my amazing entity-clearing buddy and loving friend.

Thank you, Eram Saeed: you trained me to be an amazing telesummit speaker, and thanks to you, I have an amazing, loving, Sensitive Soul tribe!

Thank you, Dr. Eldon Taylor, Penney Peirce, Dr. Bruce Lipton, Lion Goodman, Tyhson Banighen, Caroline Cory, Diana Kushenbach, and Gregg Braden: learning from you has revolutionized my way of thinking and perceiving the world. I'm so very grateful.

Thank you, Marcus Bird, Kimberley Banfield, Quinn Hand, and all the mentors, staff, and students in the Wellness Leadership Academy: your expert mentoring and support has saved me years of struggling on my own. Your systems have revolutionized my business and my ability to deliver my *magic*. Thank you for accepting my woo-woo-ness and for continuing to cheer me on.

Thank you, Andy Ramsay: for sharing your kick-ass off- and online expertise, and for helping me understand how to apply the principles of quantum physics for masterful manifesting in my everyday life.

Thank you, Cathy Hohmeyer: for being my healer "bestie" and for always introducing me to new stuff to expand my understanding, awareness, and consciousness!

Thank you, Jack and Joan Devitt: for believing in me so many years ago, even though I didn't believe in myself. Your loving support and guidance have given me peak moments in my life.

Thank you, Bob Kavanaugh: you introduced the world of aliens to me, helped me see the big picture, and offered your support and friendship.

Thank you, Mimi Wacholder, Marc Fenczak, and Karen Courtland-Kelly: you helped me express my love and light through the sport of figure skating.

Thank you, Meg Parker, Gretchen Lansing, Rebecca Wolford, DL Walker, and Drs. Joseph and Rhiannon Clauss: for rebalancing my body when it needs some hands-on TLC, so I can keep doing what I love doing.

Thank you to all my joint venture partners, especially Jeff Gignac and Isa Herrera, and my amazing LifeWave team members, friends, and colleagues, and those who have supported my work and mission throughout the years. Because of you, this book will impact a lot more people.

Thank you, Darius Barazandeh, Ian Shelley, and Tammy Mastroberte for letting me share my magic with your beautiful Sensitive Soul communities.

Thank you, David Schmidt: your phototherapy patches helped me go from the depths of illness and despair years ago to becoming the gold-medal winning Energizer Bunny® I am today! Thanks to your brilliant anti-aging technology, I am healthier now than I was two decades ago. Your friendship and continued support are priceless.

Thank you, Dr. Yury Kronn, Galina Kalyuzhny, Yvonne Angeletti, Lorina Millard, and the whole Energy Tools International team for making my dreams come true by doing the R&D and infusing Ascension 3 frequencies into my jewelry line!

Thank you to my ex-partner, Sean Guenette, who modeled self-trust and self-reliance. You pushed me to become strong and fearless. Because of you, I am now a multi-gold-winning medalist in adult figure skating in three disciplines.

Thank you to my amazing team: Tasha Lesiak, Taylor Price, Cecilia Santos, Jake Kent, Anna Izzo Rissberger, Bronwyn Seal, Tanya Graves, and Jackie Miller. People often wonder how I can juggle all these balls at once, and it's because of the amazing work you do behind the scenes. I love you guys!

Thank you to my family, who has supported me through all the radical changes that have occurred in my life due to my unconventional choices. Your love and patience over the years have given me a solid foundation from which to grow and take flight.

Thank you to my *Sensitive Soul kids*, with whom I've had the privilege to teach and work. My time with you is precious, and I'm so thrilled to see how you are growing and evolving! I'm honored to be chosen as (Fairy) Godmother to Camaya.

Thank you to my accountability partner, Sandi Goldi, who meets with me every Monday morning, so we can share our wins, our challenges, and our commitments. It's been an honor and pleasure to watch our paths grow and evolve.

Thank you to my Light Warrior tribe, my students and clients: your love and support mean the world to me. We're healing the world together one day at a time, and I'm so very grateful for your light.

Thank you to my partner, James P. Gann: you've been the muscle behind my mission. Being the busy bee that I am, I can relax knowing you've always got my back. You're the fun maestro who gets me up and moving whenever I'm too glued to the computer. You and our dog, Apache, are a constant source of love, light, and laughs. You're my rock at home so that I can be the rock star out there.

Thank you to my God Team: you've been patient with my stubbornness over the years and I'm delighted and grateful that I can feel your loving presence and guidance in my life every day. I am so blessed!

Lastly, thank you to my readers. I know that reading this book has the potential to ignite your inner gifts, so you can shine your light brighter. The world needs your light. Thank you for trusting in me as your guide.

Introduction

YOU ARE *NOT* THE PROBLEM

Are you highly sensitive? If you are, you're in the right place. If you've been told that it's a bad thing, I'm here to tell you it is not. Before I go on, here's a quiz you can take to see if you fit the description of a highly sensitive person. Tally how many *yes* answers you have from this list:

- ☐ Do you see yourself as an empath or have you been labeled as being *too sensitive*?

- ☐ Are you highly intuitive, creative, imaginative, artistic, love colors or crystals?

- ☐ Are you an expert at anticipating another person's needs or wants?

- ☐ Are you more comfortable in nature than you are in a bustling city?

- ☐ Do you often get weird or unusual side effects from traditional medications or find they do not work for you?

- ☐ Are you negatively affected by watching pain and violence depicted in the news, in shows, or in movies?

- ☐ Are you able to see, hear, feel, or sense things that other people can't, even as a child (imaginary friends, angels, ghosts)?

- ☐ Do you get drained and overwhelmed in crowds, cities, or shopping malls and avoid negative people because you tend to absorb their emotions like a sponge?

☐ Have you developed one or more of the following: fibromyalgia, adrenal fatigue, autoimmune disease, or multiple environmental or chemical sensitivities?

☐ Have you been diagnosed with agoraphobia, generalized or social anxiety, ADHD (attention deficit hyperactivity disorder), or ASD (autism spectrum disorder)?

If you said yes to three or more questions, you are likely someone I call a *Sensitive Soul.*

According to research by Dr. Elaine N. Aron, up to 30 percent of the population is highly sensitive.[1] In her work, she discusses a sensitive's depth of processing, overstimulation, emotional responsivity or empathy, and sensitivity to subtleties. I'm in that 30 percent, and maybe you are too.

When I was growing up, I had a hard time fitting in with other school children. I was kind and gentle with everyone, especially the children in my class who at that time were labeled *mentally retarded.* They were being bullied for being *stupid,* and I was being bullied for being sweet, smart, and soft-spoken. But because my family was religious and because I was terrified of conflict, I never fought back. My younger siblings had to rescue me one day when the neighbor's kids thought it would be fun to choke me with my own winter scarf because I wouldn't fight back.

As a highly sensitive child, I worried all the time about other people. I could feel other people's pain and sadness. I wanted to help but didn't know how. I couldn't watch the news without almost bursting into

1 F. Lionetti et al. "Dandelions, Tulips, and Orchids: Evidence for the Existence of Low-Sensitive, Medium-Sensitive, and High-Sensitive Individuals in the General Population." *Translational Psychiatry.* (2018) 8(1):24. europepmc.org/article/PMC/5802697

tears. I wanted to rescue everyone who was suffering in the world, and I felt a huge burden on my shoulders.

When you were growing up, did you feel that way?

Not once while I was growing up did an adult say to me, "Your sensitivity is a *good* thing. It's a gift." I grew to believe that my sensitivity was a curse, something I'd learn to overcome by becoming stronger and tougher.

"Grow a thicker skin!" my first husband would say to me.

But try as I might, I couldn't do it. I couldn't *not* feel people's stuff. It was my nature. I felt trapped and overwhelmed by my sensitivity. I wanted so much to be someone other than me. I asked God to *fix me*—to make me stronger. I daydreamed about becoming a superhero, so I could put the bullies in their place, rescue the suffering, and save the world.

There is a saying in Chinese that makes fun of people who are sensitive. They call us *tofu*. Highly sensitive people are labeled tofu because, like this food, we are soft and easily crumbled. My mom is highly sensitive, and we both grew up being made fun of because we were tofu.

Now I know that sensitivity isn't a problem; it's a gift.

Signs that my sensitivity could be useful came when I started medical school. Because I was highly empathic, I could feel what my patients needed—I knew exactly what their fears were, and thus, could counsel them in a way that made them feel respected and heard.

I began unconsciously tapping in to my sensitivity to help make medical diagnoses. I clearly remember one case in which a fourteen-year-old boy came into the hospital with abdominal pain. He looked scared and almost paralyzed from pain. The first thought I had was *appendicitis*, so I asked all the right questions and did the right physical exam to confirm the diagnosis. I immediately contacted the surgeon on call and told her I had a patient with appendicitis who needed surgery.

The surgeon examined the boy and ran some lab tests and scans. The lab results came back with a normal white blood cell count, and the scans were inconclusive. She wanted to wait before doing surgery because he didn't have a high white blood cell count. I started getting a bit antsy but realized we had to wait for parental consent, so I let a few hours go by before bugging the surgeon again. After hours had passed, I called the surgeon again, almost begging her to do the surgery.

Finally, she agreed. Her gut was telling her that the labs didn't reflect how this child looked. Sure enough, when she did the surgery, she found a huge abscess walling off a burst appendix. After surgery, the patient's white blood cell count skyrocketed, as expected with appendicitis. He felt sicker than before the surgery, but he survived and made a full recovery. Had the surgeon waited longer, the abscess might have broken open, risking blood poisoning and death.

As a medical doctor, being super-sensitive came in handy on many occasions. However, I felt drained because I didn't know how to manage my gift. By the time I was in my early thirties, my body broke down from the massive stress of feeling too much. I ended up with fibromyalgia, chronic fatigue syndrome, depression, and autoimmunity. I developed the same symptoms as my mother had when she became disabled in her forties.

At the time, I didn't understand the connection between my symptoms and my sensitivity. I thought I was weak. With my self-esteem running at an all-time low, I cried myself to sleep each night. I wanted to die. I felt like a failure. Somehow, I had expected myself to be perky and happy all the time, especially at work. Even my staff figured out that something was wrong, despite my pretending to be okay.

I felt shame about going on partial disability. I felt guilty for not being as solid as a rock for my patients, family, and friends. I felt completely lost and overwhelmed.

But here's the good part.

My illness slowed me down enough for me to contemplate the meaning of life. I was having an existential crisis, or as the spiritual folks say, a *Dark Night of the Soul*. I hit rock bottom. One night, while crying myself to sleep, I heard an inner voice say: *You have a choice.*

That was the turning point in my miserable life.

Somehow, I got the courage to divorce my husband and make a new life for myself, despite being partially disabled and having a mountain of debt.

I connected with a local Reiki Master spiritual teacher, Pat, and she helped me heal spiritually and emotionally. My body healed quickly, and I recovered from my major illnesses within two years—something unheard of in conventional medicine.

Thanks to my spiritual counselor and teacher, I learned to harness my sensitivity as a gift instead of admonishing myself for it. Through years of studying energy medicine and spiritual healing, I tapped my sensitivity as a gift. What's more, I began to use it as a Superpower. I learned to control my sensitivity so I wouldn't be overwhelmed by other people's energy. I learned I could use my intuitive information to help my patients, clients, students, friends, and family members.

I discovered I could also utilize my sensitivity to send healing energy remotely to others and to influence the weather. I would converse with and send healing to people who were in a coma due to trauma. They would wake up suddenly, astounding doctors with their speed of recovery. Instead of being a burden, my sensitivity became an asset, helping me with making important life decisions.

After years of learning how to harness my sensitivity as a Superpower, I feel compelled to share what I've learned with the world. Why? Because there are countless sensitive people suffering when they could be thriving. If every kind, sensitive person could use their gifts, shine their light, and fulfill their purpose, the world would be a happier place.

Wouldn't you agree?

If you or a loved one is a highly Sensitive Soul, it's time to learn how to harness that sensitivity as a Superpower. Read on, and I'll show you how you can become a superhero in your own life.

Chapter 1

World Sensitivity Crisis

WHAT'S HAPPENING WITH SENSITIVE PEOPLE

A 2015 meta-analysis of 175 worldwide studies on ADHD (attention deficit hyperactivity disorder) in children found the prevalence of ADHD was approximately 7.2 percent of the general population.[2] In the United States, that number was 10.2 percent, according to another study that ended in 2016.[3]

The number of women diagnosed and medicated for adult ADHD has increased 344 percent in one decade, according to a Center for Disease Control and Prevention report.[4]

In 2012, doctors Scott Hayter and Matthew Cook published a study covering 81 autoimmune diseases, and estimated prevalence in the United States at about 14.7 million.[5]

2 Rae Thomas et al. "Prevalence of Attention-Deficit/Hyperactivity Disorder: A Systematic Review and Meta-analysis." *Pediatrics.* (April 2015). 135(4), pp. e994–e1001.
3 Xu Guifeng et al. "Twenty-Year Trends in Diagnosed Attention-Deficit/Hyperactivity Disorder Among US Children and Adolescents." *JAMA Netw Open.* 2018 Aug 3;1(4):e181471. pubmed.ncbi.nlm.nih.gov/30646132
4 Kayla N. Anderson et al. "Attention-Deficit/Hyperactivity Disorder Medication Prescription Claims Among Privately Insured Women Aged 15–44 Years — United States, 2003–2015." *MMWR Morb Mortal Wkly Rep.* January 19, 2018, 67(2);66–70. cdc.gov/mmwr/volumes/67/wr/mm6702a3.htm
5 Hayter, Scott M. and Matthew C. Cook. "Updated Assessment of the Prevalence, Spectrum and Case Definition of Autoimmune Disease." *Autoimmun Rev.* 2012 Aug;11(10):754–65. pubmed.ncbi.nlm.nih.gov/22387972

According to the World Health Organization, one in four people will experience a mental or neurological disorder during their lifetime.[6] Depression is the leading cause of disability around the world.

While the rest of the world clamors to resolve the shortage of a variety of drugs to address these problems, I'm here to offer a different perspective. Although pharmaceutical drugs can be lifesaving in emergencies and supportive for symptom relief for several acute and chronic conditions, they don't address the issues that may be underlying someone's susceptibility to certain illnesses.

In my experience as a medical doctor and as one who works almost exclusively with highly sensitive people, I've come to the realization that our quick-fix society has been medicating the common symptoms associated with being highly sensitive, instead of learning how to mitigate them using conscious awareness and training. The symptoms of ADHD and autoimmunity are extremely common among highly sensitive people, more so than for the average person.

In 1952, there were 106 mental health disorders listed in the DSM I— the very first *Diagnostic and Statistical Manual of Mental Disorders*—the manual psychiatrists use to diagnose and treat mental illness. By 2013, the DSM V listed 297 mental disorders. More children than ever are being medicated for depression and anxiety. Few, if any, of these drugs have been proven in studies to be safe for children. Furthermore, many of these drugs pose a suicide risk in children and teens.[7]

It's common in the United States for school-aged children to be evaluated for ADHD, and many parents comply with suggestions to put their children on long-term medication without so much as a blink of an eye. Some teachers I've worked with who believe medicating

6 who.int/whr/2001/en/

7 Madeline Levin et al. "Do Antidepressants Increase Suicide Attempts? Do They Have Other Risks?" *National Center for Health Research.* (n.d.) center4research.org/antidepressants-increase-suicide-attempts-risks/

children with symptoms is not appropriate are not permitted to suggest lifestyle changes—such as sugar avoidance, meditation, and electromagnetic radiation protection—because those are considered outside the teachers' area of expertise. However, every child I've seen with ADHD symptoms is highly sensitive to energy. That means their bodies become stressed due to a variety of environmental stimuli, among them: fluorescent lights, computers, Wi-Fi, food additives and colorings, excessive sugar, heavy metals, and emotional stress.

Some of these children are lucky, however, and their parents do their own research and do not take pill-popping lightly. One teen in my practice was having great difficulty in school. His grades were plummeting, and he was moody and uncooperative. "Todd" and his parents were being pressured to medicate him with ADHD drugs. His parents came to me, asking if there were alternatives.

Recognizing his extreme sensitivity to a variety of energies, I advised the parents to clean up his diet by feeding him whole foods; avoiding artificial colorings, additives, and mercury-laden tuna fish; adding a few supplements based on his symptoms; and using energy protection devices to decrease the negative effects of EMF pollution on his body. Pretty soon, Todd began acting like a normal, healthy teen. His grades rose, he completed high school with honors, and he is currently working outdoors in the wild where he belongs.

Beyond lifestyle changes and environmental manipulation, there are so many other ways to help highly sensitive and gifted people. The purpose of this book is to show you these other ways, so you can thrive in a world full of disharmonious energies.

This book distills much of the training we do at a live event called *The Light Warrior Training Camp*. In the next chapter, I summarize the benefits and limitations of the support currently available to Sensitive Souls.

Chapter 2

Sensitivity Support

WHATEVER YOU'VE TRIED ISN'T WORKING

The current solution to sensitivity symptoms involves several strategies, some lesser known than others:

1. Mitigating physical symptoms with medications
2. Stress management and counseling
3. Naturopathic and functional (lifestyle) medicine to restore and optimize the body's resiliency and health
4. Energy medicine modalities to rebalance the body's energy field
5. Environmental manipulation and remediation

Let's explore each item so you can understand the benefits and limitations of each strategy.

MEDICATIONS

Today's pharmaceutical medications are either synthetic substances or natural substances mutated to become new patentable substances that have been proven in at least two clinical studies to be more effective than placebos in mitigating symptoms associated with specific diseases or conditions. In my experience as a medical doctor, the benefits of pharmaceutical medications include the numbing of sensitivity symptoms.

Antidepressants, although known to be a suicide risk for youth, have been popularized ever since the release of the first non-drowsy antidepressant, Prozac. My mother tried this medication for her depression. At first, we thought it was going to be the miracle drug we prayed for. Unfortunately, when she stopped it suddenly, she experienced severe anxiety, withdrawal symptoms, and suicidal thoughts. Thinking it was just her disease getting worse, she was placed on another drug. It wasn't until years later, when she was using phototherapy patches over specific acupuncture points to help her symptoms of hives, that we discovered the patches caused her depression symptoms to subside. She was finally able to wean herself off antidepressants for good.

Antipsychotic drugs are used when people have hallucinatory symptoms, including seeing and hearing things other people can't see or hear. Some people clearly require these drugs simply to function before they can safely pursue other healing modalities and strategies. That being said, I have met highly Sensitive Souls who can *hear* conversations from other realities, including nonhuman ones, and those who can *see* spirits, aliens, and other timelines. These can be challenging cases to deal with and require skills beyond what can be taught in a book, but I want to let you know not everyone labeled *psychotic* is mentally ill. They may just be extremely and indiscriminately sensitive to energies.

Sedatives and hypnotic drugs are habit-forming but are unfortunately prescribed to many Sensitive Souls who cannot sleep at night because they are aware of too much, even in their sleep. Unable to escape the cycle of addiction and insomnia, they stay on these medications, despite the lack of safety data on long-term use, because their doctors don't offer any other option. That puts them at risk for liver, kidney, and possibly brain damage.

STRESS MANAGEMENT AND COUNSELING

Whether from prayer, meditation, mindfulness, or walking in nature, everyone can benefit from stress management skills. The problem, unfortunately, is that these skills are not taught to conventional medical practitioners. As a result, they are then ill-equipped to teach it to their patients. Furthermore, medical insurance companies often do not reimburse doctors adequately for spending time counseling or coaching their patients, so there is less of an incentive to do so.

For example, one of the local doctors in my town could routinely see up to sixty patients a day, and he happened to be the top prescriber of narcotics according to other nurses and providers in the area. It wasn't that he wanted to prescribe narcotics to people in chronic pain. He didn't know what else to do with these patients, especially since the average doctor visit was five to ten minutes long.[8] I, on the other hand, could only manage to see fifteen to twenty people a day in my office when I was a practicing family physician, because I was dedicated to counseling and coaching my patients. I wrote few narcotic scripts, so drug-seekers didn't bother to get on my schedule.

Because I could not compete with the number of patients seen per day, the hospital I worked for told me they were going to cut my salary, despite the fact that I mainly saw underprivileged poor people who were suffering from many chronic diseases, unlike their much healthier, educated counterparts in the resort town one hour away.

Health practitioners are supposed to model wellness for their patients, and in many ways, they do. Many practitioners I know in my small town eat food from farmers' markets and exercise regularly. Unfortunately, the grand majority are still stressed because of their work situation: constant pressure from their employers to see more patients, student

---

8 Greg Irving et al. "International variations in primary care physician consultation time: a systematic review of 67 countries." *BMJ Open*. Volume 7, Issue 10. bmjopen.bmj.com/content/7/10/e017902

debt, sick and dying patients, insurance companies, on-call duties, and so on. Few, if any, practice meditation or mindfulness on a regular basis. And that was true of me until very recently.

How can we expect patients to manage their stress if their healthcare providers themselves can't do it?

Working with a counselor or coach is a wonderful way for Sensitive Souls to feel heard and honored. Talking with a trained, nonjudgmental counselor can help us feel safer and more connected. Counseling may fail, however, when highly sensitive people share their extreme and unusual symptoms—like being able to see ghosts—and the counselor assumes they are exhibiting a mental illness rather than a Superpower gift. The fear, of course, is obtaining a one-way ticket to the psychiatric ward and being pumped full of antipsychotic drugs.

NATUROPATHIC AND FUNCTIONAL MEDICINE

I'm a big fan of naturopathic and functional medicine because both specialties understand that our lifestyle choices are of the utmost importance in health and wellness.

Naturopathic doctors, or NDs, receive separate training from medical doctors. Naturopaths focus on wellness and restoring the body's physical health through nutrition, lifestyle, stress management, and natural remedies. They know how to balance the body so it heals from within, rather than relying on pharmaceutical drugs or surgery.

Some, but not all, functional medical practitioners are medical doctors or MDs. Some are nutritionists, for example. Those who are medical doctors are trained additionally outside the conventional medical system and are sometimes considered rogue doctors by their peers. However, the number of celebrity functional medicine specialists is growing, with many authoring bestselling books. They are turning the tide on the prevailing attitude toward functional medicine practitioners. They are becoming more mainstream among wellness enthusiasts.

Whether or not you are a Sensitive Soul, proper rest, nutrition, exercise, stress management, and restorative practices are vital to wellness and health. If you are not already well-versed in the philosophy of food as medicine, then I highly recommend you read up on how to revitalize your health using good nutrition as a foundation. The average citizen and many governments are decades behind the times when it comes to the science of healthy nutrition. If you're not reading current books or watching documentaries about it, you're probably getting the wrong information.

In the book, *Demand Better! Revive Our Broken Health Care System* (Second River Healthcare Press, March 2011) by Sanjaya Kumar, chief medical officer at Quantros; and David B. Nash, dean of the Jefferson School of Population Health at Thomas Jefferson University; the authors reveal that only a fraction of treatments doctors commonly recommend have been subjected to high-quality research or have been proven as effective and safe.

Although it is wonderful to have a naturopathic or functional medicine practitioner in your corner, few are equipped to show highly sensitive people how to clear themselves of other people's negative emotional energy or how to use their sensitivity gifts to produce a healing effect on a loved one 3,000 miles away. These are some of the skills you'll learn from this book.

ENERGY MEDICINE MODALITIES

Energy medicines, both new and old, powerfully affect the subtle energy flowing in, through, and around our bodies. In Traditional Chinese Medicine, it is taught that energetic imbalances underlie all chronic physical illnesses. Until our energy is balanced, the physical illness will not fully heal.

In scientific terms, energetic balance is an invisible blueprint that forms the scaffolding for building the physical body. For example, if the energetic blueprint for making a healthy liver was unhealthy and unbalanced, every liver cell produced would become unhealthy as well. Given the rapid turnover of cells in our bodies, it's said we grow a brand-new body every seven to ten years.

Then why, you may ask, do people's organs and cells keep degenerating as we age, rather than being replaced by healthy young cells? The answer is in the blueprint, also known as a *morphic field*. If the field is unhealthy, the organs and cells will be unhealthy.

The value of energy medicine and modalities, such as qigong, Reiki, healing touch, and acupuncture, is that they can rebalance your energy field when practiced regularly and with consciousness. These therapies and techniques can be extremely supportive to highly sensitive people because their energetic systems are often overwhelmed.

One way some energetic medicine modalities are weak is in dealing with spiritual and dimensional imbalances. Although most deal with Spirit, Sensitive Souls deal with spiritual imbalances that are not healable through these means. Dimensional imbalances—imbalances traced to other dimensions and other nonhuman dimensional beings—are beyond what we can talk about in this book, but I teach students how to deal with them in a training program found in my Academy of Light Medicine.

In this book, I show simple and effective energy clearing and balancing techniques specifically designed for highly sensitive people so they can feel more relaxed, stable, and grounded every day.

ENVIRONMENTAL MANIPULATION
AND REMEDIATION

Many highly sensitive people have already discovered that to function, they must live their lives differently from most non-sensitive people. That means wearing sunglasses and ear plugs when they go into a supermarket or in a crowd. It means living in the country instead of the city. It means having a Wi-Fi-free, smartphone-free home. It means sleeping on a grounding mat or *earthing*—bare skin touching the earth—outside every day. Or it may mean avoiding family or friends who are energy vampires or toxic energy influences.

By the time highly sensitive people find me, they've already been estranged from many of their loved ones. They are outcasts in their own family. No one understands them, and their greatest wish is to be *normal*. They've done everything they can think of to manipulate and remediate their environment so that they aren't suffering as much from their sensitivity, but life is hard.

One of the first things I tell them is their sensitivity isn't a curse, it is a gift that they haven't yet learned to control. Although training your gifts isn't an overnight process, I guarantee that once you learn to manage them—rather than them managing you—your life will be more miraculous and wondrous than ever before.

In the next chapter, I share the Sensitivity-to-Superpower Formula, a way in which you can start turning your sensitivity gift into an asset you can use to experience more ease, more fun, and more miracles! Are you ready?

Let's do this!

Chapter 3

The Sensitivity-to-Superpower Formula

IT'S TIME TO OWN YOUR SUPERPOWERS

The skills you train through this book might at first seem impossible or, at least, improbable. If you've already skimmed through the Contents you might be asking the following questions: *Me? Influence the weather? Who do you think I am? Storm from the comic book, X-men? Aw, c'mon, you've got to be kidding me, right? I'm not that great. I'm not that gifted.*

Let me ask you this: why *not* you?

Every Sensitive Soul I've met is highly gifted, without exception. It's a matter of changing your perspective to honor your sensitivity as a gift, rather than a curse. Once you've at least considered that possibility, we can get to work on making life fun and enjoyable for you.

First things first. Let me show you what we'll be doing in this book—something I call the Sensitivity-to-Superpower Formula.

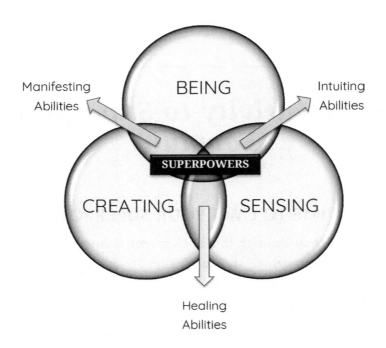

The first step in owning your gift is to own your energy. That means getting to know the real *you* on a vibratory level. To take control of your gifts, you must vibrate at your core level of BEING. It is only from this state you can master and evolve all your gifts.

In Penney Peirce's book, *Frequency*, the author describes how each of us has our own unique vibration, our Home Frequency. I have found when we resonate at our home frequency, we are in alignment with our highest selves, and we feel peaceful and positive, regardless of our outer circumstances.

Once you've begun practicing BEING you, you can progress to using your natural gift of SENSING. Highly sensitive people already have heightened senses, so it won't be difficult to waken up your *inner senses*—those beyond your five regular senses of seeing, touching, tasting, hearing, and smelling.

You'll be able to sense and gather information using your inner senses of *clairvoyance, clairsentience, clairgustience, clairaudience, clairessence,* or *claircognizance.* I call these your *clairs.* You will naturally have one that is dominant. You can discover which one by noticing how you talk and how you interact with the world. You can also figure it out through your symptoms, if you have any.

For example, if someone asks you if you understand something they've said, you might answer, *I see what you mean* (clairvoyance), or *I hear you* (clairaudience), or *I feel you* (clairsentience). You may answer differently at different times, which may mean that although you most likely have a dominant clair, you have access to many more.

If physical symptoms seem to be at the forefront of your awareness, you are likely clairsentient-dominant. If hearing voices, even inside your mind, is a common occurrence, then you're most likely clairaudient-dominant. If you are able to see spirits or someone's aura, or you often see pictures in your mind, you're likely clairvoyant-dominant. Most people have one of these three as their dominant inner sense.

Claircognizance, also known as *clairknowing,* is the one clair that everyone wants to have on lock. It's the ability to know Divine truth without the physical proof.

Many people experience intuition as a gut feeling. Sometimes this feeling is reactive; sometimes this feeling is downright uncomfortable. I remember the time I first met my current husband at a park, 3,000 miles from my home. I had been consciously manifesting my ideal love partner for months, yet I had no clue this man I met at the park was *him.* Hours after I met him, I experienced extreme abdominal pain for seemingly no reason.

I didn't realize until months later that my body had been trying to tell me to pay attention—that this man would be my future husband. It was a painful intuitive hit.

In Dr. Mona Lisa Schulz's book, *Awakening Intuition*, she describes an incident of clairknowing that I'll never forget. Her mother was having dinner with her father, geographically far removed from where Mona Lisa lived. All of a sudden, Mona Lisa's mother stood up, turned to her father and said, matter-of-factly, "Mona Lisa is in trouble." At that moment, thousands of miles away, Mona Lisa was hit by a truck. Talk about mother's intuition!

One thing that impresses me about this story is how calm her mother was. When we think we've had an intuitive hit, but we're scared, the hit is likely inaccurate. Our egoic fears and prejudices cloud accurate intuition most of the time.

It's one thing to have unconscious intuitive hits, like those I just described, and a whole other thing to be able to consciously access intuitive information at will. Wouldn't you like to be able to get accurate answers to all your pressing questions in an instant, rather than have to wait for intuitive hits to drop in randomly?

In the chapters that follow, I explain different methods of gaining intuitive information with greater precision and ease. When you are consciously BEING and consciously SENSING, not only will you get full access to your intuiting abilities, but you'll increase your accuracy by a long shot. Isn't that cool?

The remainder of this book is divided into the three sections of BEING, SENSING, and CREATING. After discussing BEING and SENSING in this book, we discuss CREATING. In the CREATING chapters, you will use your intention and imagination to create a New Reality from the one you're currently in. By SENSING and CREATING, you'll maximize your healing abilities. Not only that, but you'll be able to manipulate your reality, *including the weather*.

Don't worry your ego will grow too big to handle. Most highly sensitive people I've met have been through so much self-loathing and self-criticism at various points in their lives that they need to experience their own power to change their reality. If you can change the weather to your liking and for the highest good, what more will you be able to change in your own life?

By BEING while you are CREATING, you'll be able to connect to your Divine Path and fully access your manifesting abilities. BEING at your home frequency more and more (I'll share with you the magic number of how much is ideal later) while consciously SENSING and CREATING is the way toward Superpower Mastery in all areas of your life.

How exciting!

In the BEING section, you learn to connect with the highest form of Inner Guidance, also known as *Source, Creator, God, Zero Point, Stillness, The Void, The Divine,* and *The Universe.* This is the starting point for honing, managing, and expressing your Superpowers. Using a specific technique for highly sensitive people called STOIM, *Stillness Through Observing Internal Movement,* you can quickly and easily move into a state of perpetual peace, as well as dissolve uncomfortable negative emotions. In this section, you'll learn *Divine Muscle Testing,* a technique you can use to receive immediate Divine Guidance through your physical body, as well as how to extract your foundational Soul Mission, or Soul Purpose, via the *Soul Mission Matrix.* Even after thousands of healing sessions I've conducted, I am still in awe of how powerful it is for the client to understand their Soul Purpose with clarity.

In the second section of this book, the SENSING section, you tap your intuitive Superpowers. Here, you begin your training in *Transformational Telepathy,* a simple but powerful way to use your intuitive skills for one-way communicating with others to shift the quality of relationships. Next, you develop the skills to overcome any obstacle in your life with Perception Kung Fu. Then, you hone your sensing, intuitive skills through *Intuitive Impressioning*, a handy technique you can use to make life decisions with greater ease and speed. It can also be used to accurately read into the likes, preferences, and emotions of a person with whom you have a relationship, to better understand and empathize with them. *Healing by Proxy-Prop* is a safe way to perform a type of remote hands-on healing, on yourself or others, that doesn't require years of face-to-face training or certification. In my live events, even newbies to energy healing were able to achieve results from performing this technique on their volunteer subjects right away, much to their utter amazement.

We have some real fun in Section 3, the CREATING section. Here you learn *Travel Magic*, *Weather Magic*, and *Transmutational Bubble Magic*, in which you imagine new possibilities in your mind and create new realities in your life. *Sensitive Soul SOS™ Clearing* techniques assist you in clearing and grounding energies from your energy field that are negative, harmful, or draining. And, by the way, if you've ever dreamed of *telekinesis*—moving things with your mind—then you're going to love the chapter on *Cloud Sculpting*. The Nirvana of No chapter will help you with healthy boundaries, a crucial skill for Sensitive Souls.

In the CREATING section, I also show you how to effectively manifest any positive desires in your life using STOIM for Masterful Manifesting.

Regardless of the trials and turmoil you may have experienced in the past, I encourage you, a highly sensitive person, to see yourself now as being gifted rather than cursed, free rather than trapped, and powerful rather than insufferable. I am over-the-top excited that you are embarking on this journey with me and so many other sensitives.

Let's harness those Superpowers, shall we?

SECTION 1

BEING

Chapter 4

STOIM

THE GATEWAY TO YOUR SUPERPOWERS

You've probably heard that meditation is good for you. And there are a lot of data supporting that.

In a study by Killingsworth and Gilbert, an iPhone app was used to track self-reported happiness scores of 2,250 volunteers.[9] The app contacted 2,250 volunteers at random intervals to ask how happy they were, what they were currently doing, and whether they were thinking about their current activity or about something else that was pleasant, neutral, or unpleasant. The results were quite intriguing. "Mind-wandering is an excellent predictor of people's happiness," Killingsworth concluded. "In fact, how often our minds leave the present and where they tend to go is a better predictor of our happiness than the activities in which we are engaged." In this study, mind-wandering was a predictor of lowered happiness.

In another study, Richard Davidson, professor of psychology and psychiatry at the University of Wisconsin School of Medicine and Public Health, demonstrated significant changes to the emotional centers of the brain with meditation.[10] After volunteers were instructed on a simple meditation technique, Davidson found that

---

9 Killingsworth, Matthew A. and Daniel T. Gilbert. "A Wandering Mind Is an Unhappy Mind." *Science*. Nov. 12, 2010 330:932. danielgilbert.com/KILLINGSWORTH%20&%20GILBERT%20(2010).pdf
10 Goleman, Daniel, and Richard J. Davidson. Altered Traits: *Science Reveals How Meditation Changes Your Mind, Brain, and Body*. Avery, 2017.

the brain activity increased in areas of the brain related to attention and decision-making but became less emotionally reactive to stressful stimuli (such as a screaming baby). "Most people, if they heard a baby screaming, would have some emotional response," Davidson says, but not the highly experienced meditators. "They do hear the sound, we can detect that in the auditory cortex, but they don't have the emotional reaction."

Experienced meditators who practiced over 40,000 hours of meditation showed minimal changes to the brain while exposed to stressful stimuli. "There was a brief increase in activity as they started meditating, and then it came down to baseline, as if they were able to concentrate in an effortless way."

When I learned about this, I thought I'd better start meditating. I have to be honest, though. I was not a fan of long meditation sessions. I was too busy. I did not resonate with sitting for thirty, forty, sixty minutes at a time, meditating. It was very difficult to still my mind. I tried all sorts of techniques, but I got frustrated. Sadly, I kept thinking about my to-do list.

My spiritual teachers told me meditation was important. But I'm a results-oriented person, and that means if I don't get results from what I'm doing—especially if I'm spending a lot of time doing it—I tend not to do it. Makes sense, right? Every one of my friends who meditated with any regularity didn't seem any more peaceful, successful, or happier than I was. *So why bother?* I asked myself.

One day, I stumbled upon a book with an intriguing title: *The Secrets of Instant Healing,* by Dr. Frank Kinslow. Once I learned his quantum entrainment technique, I realized that I could self-generate the same feeling, what he calls *Eufeeling,* instantly, without effort. All I had to do was feel my body, explained in more detail below, and *BAM!* I was in Eufeeling. Just beyond Eufeeling is Stillness. I was overjoyed! Dr.

Kinslow's brilliant technique showed me a doorway to Stillness I had never encountered before, and it was heaps easier than any meditation techniques I had tried before.

Here's the cool part: You can do it while your eyes are open, while you're talking, while you're eating, or while you're working. You can experience the benefits of sitting meditation without having to sit down. I know that sounds like cheating, but all I can say is it works for me, and I get results. And by results, I mean tangible worldly results, not simply *inner peace*. Stillness is another word for *Zero Point*, the term quantum physics fans refer to when they are talking about the source of all creation. In other words, from Stillness we can consciously create our reality. More on that in Section Three of this book.

I was sharing with one of my students how revolutionary this technique is, and he told me that he wasn't using it. When I asked why he didn't resonate with it, he said that he wasn't sure he was doing it right. Given that he was highly clairsentient (feels through his body), I had to figure out how to teach him differently.

Because of his difficulty, I discovered another doorway to Stillness.

I used to be a fan of scary movies. I watched a very scary movie called *The Ring*.[11] Now, there have been remakes of the movie that are probably less scary, but this version was extremely scary. It was the first time I had seen digital imaging, which made the ghost in the movie move in strange and unnatural ways.

After watching this movie, I couldn't sleep because I was so scared. I kept seeing the same scenes in my mind over and over again. No matter what I tried—breathing exercises, meditation, mindfulness, Kundalini yoga, or progressive relaxation—nothing was allowing me to sleep. I just lay in bed wide awake for hours, until I finally fell asleep

---

11 *The Ring*. Director Gore Verbinski. 2002.

from exhaustion. This went on for three days, until my mind stopped rewinding those scenes in my head.

A few years went by. While visiting a friend who was preparing to move homes, I glanced in one of her boxes and spotted the sequel to the first movie, *The Ring Two*.[12] Instinctively, I wanted to watch it so I could see what happened after the cliffhanger ending of *The Ring*.

I said, "Can I borrow this?"

My surprised husband turned to me and said, "You've got to be kidding, right? Last time you didn't sleep for three days."

"Maybe I'll watch it. Maybe I won't," I said.

After some deliberation, I decided to brave watching the sequel. I was fully prepared to stay awake again for three days straight. I knew it was going to be scary.

Yup, while watching the sequel, I became scared out of my mind again. However, the ending did resolve in a positive way, thankfully.

Oh, boy, here we go again, I thought. *No sleep for three days.*

I lay in bed, thinking to myself: *Well, last time meditation didn't work, mindfulness didn't work, Kundalini yoga didn't work, progressive relaxation didn't work, watching my breath didn't work.*

Next, I thought: *Well, since I'm going to be awake, I might as well just be scared.*

I decided in that moment, I would be fully immersed in *being* scared. What happened next was fascinating! The moment I decided I was allowing myself to be scared, I became curious: *What does being scared feel like in my body?*

---

12 *The Ring Two*. Director Hideo Nakata. 2005.

I decided to focus my attention inside my body to discover what reactions being scared created.

Suddenly I was aware of waves upon waves of strong energy pulsing and vibrating all over my entire body. I was feeling pulses of energy all the way to my fingertips, all the way up through my head, and all the way to my toes. My heart was beating so hard I thought the bed was moving. I was fascinated by how my body was reacting to being scared. It dawned on me that moments before making this decision, I hadn't felt anything in my body because I was only focused on what I was seeing in my head.

I decided to continue observing my body being scared. And, wouldn't you know it? Within ten minutes I fell sound asleep and woke up the next day fully refreshed. Then it dawned on me: *That's what it means to be fully present.*

So many spiritual teachers talk about the power of presence, but until then, I didn't fully understand what it felt like. According to intuitive, spiritual teacher, and bestselling author Carolyn Myss, when you are present, all your energy circuits are here in present time. When all your energy is here, you can heal; you can create new realities. If you aren't fully here, you can't easily heal or create.

I am highly clairsentient. It is my dominant sensitivity gift, if you will. Thus, turning this talent inward and observing the movement and vibration in my body help me become fully present. Using just my mind, or practicing mindfulness, wasn't quite as effective.

After *The Ring* incident, I realized that for most of my waking time, I was never truly present. I rarely consciously manifested a positive future as a result. I was being reactive, not creative, to whatever came my way.

Of course, after living through that amazing and enlightening experience, I completely forgot about it. Such is human nature. When we don't have an emergency or a crisis, sometimes we forget the wisdom we recently learned. There were several months in which, while regularly practicing Stillness, I was easily attracting all manner of opportunities and abundance. Then, I got busy and forgot. My success waned. I was still taking lots of positive actions in my business and home life, but manifesting my goals became more arduous. I realized I had abandoned the practice of Stillness for months because things were going well. Our very human habit is to forget about our wellness practices when things are going well. Only when things are not going well do we scramble to help or heal ourselves.

Thankfully, I got the message loud and clear from the Universe. I preferred the ease—doing less, being more, and having more. My student asked me about a different way to get into Stillness. That's when I developed STOIM, or *Stillness Through Observing Internal Movement*. It's perfect for people who are highly empathic and who sense the world kinesthetically—through their body.

When I paid attention and focused on any bit of movement or vibration in my body, it was easy to quiet my mind and arrive at Stillness as I did all those years ago when I watched *The Ring Two*.

I shared my story about being scared and feeling inside my body. I asked my student to try finding a doorway into Stillness, to pay attention to the inside of his body, and to feel any vibration or movement—to notice it without any judgment, and see if that worked for him. Lo and behold, that did the trick. Now he is a master at STOIM and has gone on to manifest amazing things in his life, including buying his dream car and being successful in his business.

STOIM: GETTING STARTED

Like Dr. Frank Kinslow, I believe it is not necessary to sit in lotus position, eyes closed, for half an hour or more to reap the benefits of meditation. If you want to, of course, go ahead. But if you want to learn how to instantly connect to Stillness, even when you are doing something else, something I call Stillness-on-the-Fly™, I recommend learning the STOIM technique. Even advanced meditators will benefit from being able to access Stillness in every situation. Unlike other meditation practices that have you focus your mind, breath, or awareness on one thing, while avoiding all other distractions, Stillness-on-the-Fly is a way to peacefully respond to all of life's ups and downs. In athletic terms, it's equivalent to being *in the zone*.

The STOIM technique helps you to achieve a state of being in which you can access the Void, the Stillness, the Zero Point. STOIM helps you naturally release energies that aren't yours—including your negative emotions and other people's emotions—without *forcing* them out. This is very helpful, even without making an intention for healing to occur.

STOIM is quick and easy to do. Let's begin.

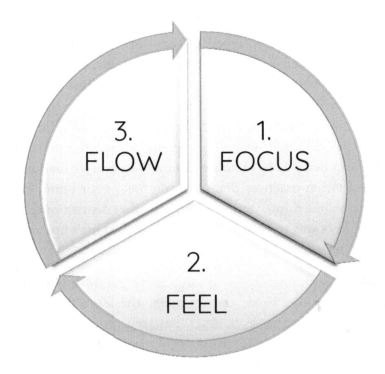

1. Initiate a movement of energy in your body that you can feel. Move the body in some way, just for a few seconds, whether rubbing your hands, stamping your feet, or dancing around the room—whatever it takes to sense energy flowing through your body.

2. Do that for a few seconds. Now stop, close your eyes, and *focus* your attention on the inside of your body.

3. Next, *feel* the movement of energy in your body. It may feel like pulsing, buzzing, or waves. Maybe you simply feel the beating of your heart.

4. Finally, follow the *flow*, the vibration of the movement inside your body. Observe it without judgment; be curious. Where do you feel the movement? Is it more on the right side or more on the left side? More on the upper half of the torso or the lower half? More on the front or the back?

Do not judge the movement; just feel it, and focus on it. That means you don't label it as *pain*. You don't label it as something *bad* or *good*; it just is what it is. You might notice that there's no flow in certain areas of your body. You can choose to pay attention to those low-flow areas on purpose, to discover what happens.

The most important point is to stay in a state of curiosity, regardless of what you're feeling or sensing.

If you're having difficulty feeling any movement, you may want to do more physical movement to elevate the energy flow in your body so your attention can be trained to feel that energy. That might mean dancing vigorously, jumping up and down, or running on the spot—whatever it takes. Then close your eyes and feel the flow. Most people find rubbing their hands together is an easy way to generate flow.

Do STOIM for a minute or so. Notice how you feel emotionally after that. Most people say when they are so focused on feeling, their emotions go to neutral. Some express a profound sense of calm. Some even feel a kind of peaceful bliss.

Even when I was in the throngs of fascination with my rapid beating heart and pulsing energy waves while scared, my emotions neutralized quickly, which is why I was able to fall asleep.

Welcome to instant inner calm and peace! ☺

Meditating on the move, what I call *Stillness-on-the-Fly*, is a fabulous way, and maybe even better way, to manage your state of being—to feel calm, peaceful, and centered, no matter what's going on around you. We talk more about why that's important in Section Three of this book, *Creating*.

Stillness-on-the-Fly is the practice of noticing the energy flowing in your body when your eyes are open and you are doing something other than sitting still trying to meditate. For example, you can be sensing your internal energy movement while typing an email, watching a movie, or doing the dishes. The only reason it is slightly more advanced than STOIM alone is because it takes practice to feel energy flow in your body when you are doing something else simultaneously. It's all about honing your attention with increasing amount of focus and precision.

The most wonderful aspect of doing Stillness-on-the-Fly is that for it to be highly beneficial, there is no minimum effective time you must focus for. In other words, doing it for seconds or minutes at a time—several times a day, whenever you think of it—is highly effective in calming your nervous system and recalibrating your energy balance. Not only that, you can apply STOIM and Stillness-on-the-Fly to any situation, stressful or not. *In my experience, a profound auto–healing state of being is produced when 9–10 percent of your waking time is connected to Stillness.* You'll also connect more easily with your intuitive abilities.

Let's take an example of what you can use STOIM for in your everyday life.

STOIM FOR NEGATIVE EMOTIONS

One of the most useful ways to employ STOIM is when you feel depressed, angry, frustrated, sad, or otherwise in a bad mood. There have been so many times when something happens in my day, and I feel anxious, afraid, or worried. If I remember in that instance to do STOIM and feel my body in whatever emotional state I'm in, that negative emotion often dissipates effortlessly.

It's not like I'm *trying* to make the negative emotion go away. Just as when I was scared, I go into focusing, feeling, and flowing, fully embodying what that emotion feels like physically. Then, the negative emotion dissipates on its own.

Occasionally, I ask for help. If the emotions are intense, I ask my guardian angels to help me. But when I remember to do STOIM, it's amazing how quickly the negative emotions dissipate.

Here's the best part: So often when we are anxious or in trouble and looking for a viable solution to our problem, we can't think straight. When we connect to Stillness, the solution arises naturally in our awareness. It's almost like turning down the noise low enough so you can hear the whispers from Source or your guardian angels.

In other words, if you don't connect to Stillness on a regular basis, you'll be doing everything in your life the hard way. I hate to say it that bluntly, but in my experience, it's true. If you want greater ease in your life, if you want greater healing, if you want things to move faster in a positive direction, then you have a vested interest in doing STOIM as often as you can throughout the day. And if you can do twenty minutes, even better.

Now you know the technique. Here's how to apply it in emotionally charged situations: Once you notice you're in a bad mood, do everything you've learned to move into Stillness through focusing, feeling, and flowing. Eventually, when you are well practiced in this and you know how to pay attention to the vibration in your body, you will not need to move your body first or even close your eyes. But if you do right now, that's completely fine.

Keenly observe any movement in your body while you're simultaneously allowing a negative emotion in this space to just *be*. Remember when I was scared and focused attention inside my body? I noticed incredibly intense sensations within it. It's safe to do this. There's nothing dangerous about it. Focusing on your body effortlessly lessens the emotional charge.

Many people are scared of feeling. If you can make peace with feeling your body and being fully present in your body, then the emotions often resolve without fanfare. *Emotion*, some people say, stands for *Energy in motion.* Often when we feel negative emotions, we resist the uncomfortable sensation—which is a way of grabbing or holding on to it—and it can't move. As the saying goes: *What we resist, persists.* This is absolutely true in my life.

But, if we're able to fully embody the moment when we're feeling a negative emotion, it will pass through as energy in motion with no need to persist. As I said before, the benefits of doing this when you're having any sort of issue or problem is that answers or solutions will often pop up from the Stillness. Some people say it's connecting with their God, Source, the Universe, or their angels. Whatever you believe it to be, it is.

When I was first training with my intuition teacher, Laura Day, author of *The Circle* and *Practical Intuition*, I used to say I wasn't very good at locating lost objects. I would get worried and anxious about locating what I had lost. The worry was getting in the way of my intuition. Although I was good at all sorts of other types of intuitive readings, finding my lost keys or purse used to be quite challenging until I started doing STOIM.

If I'm looking for my lost keys now, eventually I remember to stop the frantic search and get fully present. I do STOIM, feel my body, and within a few seconds, an image with their exact location will pop up in my mind. Then I go directly to where they are. Do this and trust an image—or words if you're more clairaudient—will pop in, over and over again, and you will find your intuition becomes instantly available, as if it's on speed-dial.

I don't worry as much now about losing things. Try STOIM for any life situation and for resolving negative emotions, and see how it works for you. If you love sitting meditation, I encourage you to do that too. Do whatever works.

Some people are really good at meditation for forty minutes at a time, but then during the rest of their day, they're anxious, worried, and scared—not connected to the source of inner wisdom, the Stillness. If you love sitting meditation, do STOIM as well, throughout the day, seconds or minutes at a time, and see how your life changes over the days, weeks, and months. You may notice increased luck, increased synchronicities, and increased abundance. I look forward to hearing your STOIM stories. Feel free to share them in my private online community group: The Light Warrior Network (link in Next Steps).

At a Light Warrior Training Camp I led at the Omega Institute, we learned that STOIM can also be helpful in relieving pain. I asked how many participants had any sort of physical pain, and about five people in the room indicated they did. I asked them to use the techniques they had learned to move into Stillness, then pay attention to that area of pain. I instructed them not to judge it but to notice the flow or lack of energy in that area. We did STOIM for approximately three minutes. I asked them to share what happened to their pain sensations. Amazingly, every person had full resolution of their pain symptoms.

By being fully present, fully embodied, and fully sensing the vibration in your body, you can relieve pain. In my experience, doing STOIM can heal multiple areas of life.

Chapter Summary

1. There are many benefits to being in Stillness, including access to inner peace and calm.

2. You do not need to spend prolonged periods of time in sitting meditation to reap the benefits of meditation.

3. STOIM is a technique that is easy to learn, especially for empathic and highly sensitive people, and it is an easy doorway to Stillness.

4. STOIM can be used to manage and resolve stress and negative emotions and can help with pain relief.

5. With practice, you can do STOIM while doing something else. We call that *Stillness-on-the-Fly*, the benefits of which permeate every aspect of your life.

6. Stillness, or Zero Point, is the place we go to when we are ready to manifest a brand-new reality.

7. Being connected to Stillness for 9–10 percent of your waking time gets you into an auto-healing state.

Chapter 5

Divine Muscle Testing

YOUR DIRECT LINE TO THE DIVINE

Many highly sensitive people have the gift of clairaudience, among other gifts. Clairaudience is the ability to hear frequencies and energies that the average person isn't paying attention to. In other words, many of these clairaudient people can hear angels and guides—even ghosts—talk.

When people have a sudden spiritual awakening whereby they can see, hear, or feel what was once hidden to them, it can be both wondrous and frightening. If the gift of clairaudience opens up suddenly for people and they begin hearing all sorts of voices, they may think they are going crazy. Some are put on antipsychotic medications or become institutionalized.

One of the difficulties with highly clairaudient people, especially if they did not learn to manage this gift as a child, is discernment. Discernment is the ability to know whose voice is speaking (in the case of clairaudience). Discernment also plays a role for highly sensitive people being able to distinguish their "stuff" from others' "stuff." What is good and not good for you? What is true and what is a lie? Your ability to determine the truth is a function of your discernment.

Divine Muscle Testing is a technique you can use to help you with discernment, so you can find out whether something or someone or some course of action is for your highest and greatest good. Sometimes being highly clairaudient and listening to your guides is not always the best answer to what you should or shouldn't do next. Here's the reason: I know this may seem like a shock to you if you've not heard this before—but there are low-vibrational or so-called *negative* spirits whose mission is to confuse, confound, and distract humans from reaching their greatest potential. In traditional religious teachings, they are called *evil spirits* or *demons*.

Ghosts are different in that they represent disembodied spirits of previously embodied humans, and sometimes they will speak as well. If you are able to hear them, it can be very confusing. Some give advice and are trying to be helpful but don't realize that their presence is draining the energy of the host they are inadvertently attached to. Ghosts are spirits who haven't crossed over "into the light," meaning that they are still interacting on our plane of existence. Some have demons attached to them, which is why they can't find what most people call "the light."

You can use Divine Muscle Testing to determine the Light Score of something or someone. The Light Score represents the current alignment with the highest Divine Light. The higher the score, the higher the alignment with Divine Light. Conversely, the lower the score, the lower the alignment with Divine Light. Demons and ghosts (also commonly referred to as Entities) tend to have Light Scores way below 50. The more malevolent entities can have a Light Score near zero.

In addition to Light Scores, there are other scoring systems, such as the Love Score and Truth Score, that I use and teach to my students in my Academy of Light Medicine.

Dealing with low-vibrational spirits is beyond what we can cover in depth in this book, but if you'd like to know more, I teach a program for how to clear yourself, your home, your environment, and your sleep realms of negative entities and alien influences. It's called the Light Warrior Bootcamp™ 2.0 and you can check it out through the links at the back of the book.

One of my former clients was experiencing pain and discomfort. She is clairaudient. One of her guides told her to take antibiotics. I found this piece of advice rather strange because after taking a brief medical history and exam, I found no reason for her to be on antibiotics, especially given the risks and side effects involved. We used Divine Muscle Testing, which revealed that this guide, or spirit posing as her guide, had a Light Score only in the 70s, which is higher than the average person, but not high enough that we'd want to take the advice of that guide. We want all of our guardian angels and guides to be a Light Score of 100 percent.

Trusting clairaudience when you're not well trained in it from childhood can be challenging. That's just one of many examples in which discernment would be very helpful, and that's one of the reasons I teach Divine Muscle Testing.

Muscle testing is a way of using your body as an intuitive tool. There are many ways to muscle test. Traditionally, muscle testing, also called *applied kinesiology*, involves two people. The practitioner, or the tester, looks for an indication of a positive or negative response to yes/no questions by pushing down on the client's outstretched arm with increasing pressure (up to two pounds). In someone whose energy is running in the correct direction—also known as *correct polarity*—the outstretched arm locks when the answer is yes. If the answer is no, the outstretched arm becomes unlocked or temporarily weak under the same force or pressure. Using muscle testing, we can derive precise answers to yes/no questions. There are also different ways of doing intuitive muscle testing on yourself, without a partner. I teach those techniques in my live events so people can discover their own answers.

Many teachers talk about muscle testing as "connecting to and getting answers from your subconscious mind," because the subconscious mind has a memory of everything that's ever happened to you in your entire lifetime. You can ask the subconscious any question and receive an answer related to everything that it has recorded. However, I've found that the subconscious mind, although useful, is also fallible. In other words, there are programs and beliefs in the subconscious mind that may interfere with the most Divinely true answer.

I call my technique *Divine Muscle Testing* because, in my method, we are not connecting with the subconscious mind, we are connecting with the Truth of Divine Source.

Can we ask any question and get a divinely true answer for every single question we ask?

No. Knowing answers to certain questions would not be for your highest and greatest good; it would not serve you or your higher purpose. For example, getting the winning lottery numbers may not be for your highest and greatest good because it may lead you down a path that is undesirable or misaligned with your Soul Purpose.

Have people tried muscle testing for lottery numbers? Yes, and I have yet to hear of someone who has been successful at winning the lottery this way. If something is not aligned with your Divine Path, then you will not get a divinely accurate answer.

There are other things that you should know about Divine Muscle Testing and receiving answers from the Divine. In addition to certain types of questions that you may not be allowed to ask, it's not a good idea to rely on Divine Muscle Testing for important life decisions such as "Should I marry John?" "Should I jump out of this airplane?" and so on. The problem is that, as humans, we have biases, opinions, and programming that can attract *leading energies*. These energies result in incorrect answers from muscle testing. Leading energies can lead you astray, even if you are a seasoned muscle tester. Furthermore, if you have a strong bias or a strong attachment to the outcome, then accurate answers may elude you. Even so, Divine Muscle Testing can be an incredibly useful tool when used appropriately.

You can use Divine Muscle Testing to check what food your body wants, for example, or what supplements to take, or which specialist would be for your highest and greatest good. You can also use it for healing purposes. My healing students and I use Divine Muscle Testing as a way to ask Source specific questions about symptoms and arrive at solutions using a method called TOLPAKAN Healing.

In TOLPAKAN Healing, we consult three main charts to ask the foundational causes of the symptoms. Mastering this skill is empowering. I do a TOLPAKAN assessment and healing on myself just about every day. Because my Divine Muscle Testing is well practiced, I can usually get through a ton of questions and healing directives in just under ten minutes.

Now for the technique.

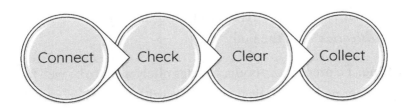

The framework of Divine Muscle Testing includes four phases:

1. *Connect*
2. *Check*
3. *Clear*
4. *Collect*

In the first phase, you ***Connect*** to Divine Source. How? Well, guess what? You've already learned how by practicing STOIM. By resonating in your BEING state, you are connected to Divine wisdom. You've already connected and opened a channel of communication by just BEING. Is that cool or what?

Within the Connect phase, a number of secondary steps make your Divine Muscle Testing even more accurate. They include connecting the energies within your physical body, so the muscle testing will be able to translate the answers consistently.

PHASE 1: CONNECT

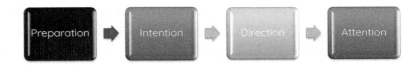

1. *Preparation* – of the body: hydrate, use Grace Point as an anchor
2. *Intention* – to connect to Divine Truth
3. *Direction* – TOLPAKAN Healing Directive
4. *Attention* – on the body

Step One: To prepare the body, you definitely want to be well hydrated because energy and electrical signals travel better when your body is hydrated. You want to anchor in your intentions, which you can do by connecting to a Grace Point found in your hand. The Grace Point is a term I learned from healers who specialize in Akashic Records Readings. I've found it to be a wonderful way to anchor the connection you've created with Divine Source. Put the thumb of one hand into the palm of the other hand, where the Grace Point is located. It's sort of like you're holding your right hand with your left hand; the left thumb is touching middle of the right palm. Some people can feel the energy emanating from the space.

Step Two: Make the *intention* to connect to the Divine Love, Light, and Truth while holding the Grace Point.

Step Three: Say the *TOLPAKAN Healing Directive*, which reinforces your intentions. It is like being the director for the play that is your reality. When you say the directive, your spiritual team is then galvanized to make it happen for you. They are there to assist you, but they don't do anything that would interfere with your soul evolution.

Here's the TOLPAKAN Healing Directive to say while connected to the Grace Point:

> *I command that I be 100 percent connected and aligned to the one and only True Source now: love, light, and truth, in the highest and best way, in all directions of time and all realities where I exist, with ease, speed, and grace. Thank you.*

Some people are hesitant to say "command" in the directives because they mistakenly liken it to the word "demand." However, the words *demand* and *command* mean two very different things. Some clients replace *command* with *request*. I advise them that, if they have such a strong aversion to the word command, they may use request; however, the energy of the statement is watered down.

The directive is really a statement: *This is the way things are going to be*, as compared with: *Could things please be like this?* Think of it as stating your future imagined reality in the NOW. Instead of *asking* for help, per se, or asking for something positive to be done, you're commanding it. Demanding would mean there's no other option; you have to have it, no matter what.

A military general commands their army. They do not make requests. Without the energy of a command, the general may not be able to lead effectively. Such is the difference in energy between the words *command*, *demand*, and *request*. Try it out for yourself. Say the directive using the word *command*, and then say it with *request*. Can you feel the difference in energy?

Step Four in the Connect phase is paying attention to your body. By paying attention to your body with great focus, you naturally go into Stillness. You also organize the energy of the body so you can be more accurate in your muscle testing.

PHASE 2: CHECK

To do the *Check* phase of Divine Muscle Testing, you'll need to choose a method of self-muscle testing.

The Body Sway Method is one of the simplest muscle-testing methods. After you've done the Connect phase, above, stand up with both feet flat on the ground and your hands at your sides.

During the Check phase of Divine Muscle Testing you'll be checking:

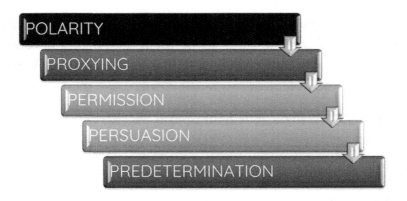

1. Is your *polarity* correct?
2. Are you *proxying*?
3. Do you have *permission* to ask this question?

4. Are there *persuasive* leading energies?
5. *Predetermine* your yes/no questions or statement.

POLARITY

The first time you muscle test, you're going to check for a yes response and a no response in your body.

1. Stand with equal weight on both your feet.
2. Keep your hands at your sides.
3. Close your eyes.
4. Say out loud to the Universe, "Show me a yes."

Wait two seconds (count *one, one thousand; two, one thousand*) and wait for your body to sway either forward or backward. If your body sways forward, then your polarity is correct. You can double check by saying, "Show me a no," and your body should gently sway backward. You don't have to do the Sway Test with your eyes closed if you feel it would be dangerous for you, but some people find they can feel subtler sway movement that way.

It's not a massive sway forward or backward that you're expecting, just a tipping movement either forward or backward. Sometimes it takes a few seconds for your body to register the response, so be patient. Once you've established that your polarity is correct, you can go to the next step and check if you are proxying.

If your polarity is incorrect, meaning that you're swaying backward when you say, "Show me a yes," or you sway forward when you say, "Show me a no," then you may have to do a polarity correction exercise. This is something that I teach during my live events.

If, while attempting the Sway Test, you do not get any motion at all, you may need to hydrate your body more. To activate energy in the body, you may need to move around a little bit. Muscle testing requires you to have balanced energy in your body. One exercise to achieve this is called the *cross-crawl*: touch your right knee to your left elbow, then your left knee to your right elbow repeatedly. Repeat about twenty times, and then try the Body Sway method again.

Some people activate the flow of *Qi*, or energy, in their body by dancing around their living room. I say do whatever works.

Some folks might feel intimidated and think they're *making* the muscle testing responses happen. This is a very adult opinion or belief; children have absolutely no problem becoming quickly proficient at muscle testing because they do not have predetermined beliefs that they can't do it.

Sitting in Stillness for a few minutes before attempting to test may be helpful for you. If you begin Divine Muscle Testing with Stillness, it will automatically make your testing much more accurate in the long run.

PROXYING

If you are *proxying* for another, that means that you are running someone else's energy in your body, whether you know it or not. Usually proxying is not something we want, but highly sensitive people seem to be at higher risk of this happening. Now this can be very, very difficult for Sensitive Souls because they can feel horrible when they're processing other people's stuff.

On a rare occasion, proxying may be necessary. It usually has to do with your Soul Mission, which you can extract for yourself using the technique shared in Chapter 6. Just know that, most of the time, it's not appropriate for people to be proxying or processing other people's stuff.

To check if you are proxying, you say your full name out loud and then wait to see whether your body sways forward or backward. For example, I would say, "My name is Karen Kan." If my polarity is correct, I should sway forward (yes). If I say a false name such as, "My name is Bob Ross," I should sway backward.

If I am proxying for another, then I will sway backward when I say, "My name is Karen Kan." In that case, I can confirm that I'm proxying by saying out loud, "My name is *not* Karen Kan," whereby I should sway forward. At times, I've had to find out who I'm proxying for because it was for the highest good. In those cases, I'll guess, using the name of something or someone that I sense might be the beneficiary of my healing energies.

The most common "others" I've proxied for are:

- Mother Earth
- Mass Consciousness
- Alternate Self
- A Soul Destiny Partner (someone whom you are responsible for helping in this or another lifetime)
- Infiniverse (all of creation)
- All of Humanity

Don't worry—when most highly sensitive people proxy, they are proxying for a person they know, such as their spouse, parent, sibling, or friend.

Most of the time, you don't need to know for whom you are proxying because it isn't appropriate, and you just need to break the proxy to get back to you. In other healing modalities, you may purposefully proxy for another and, with your muscle testing, receive answers specific to that other person with whom you have permission to heal. *Auto-proxying* is a term I invented to describe unconscious proxying for another.

Sometimes auto-proxying is appropriate, as when my energies are called forth to heal Mother Earth, for example. Other times, auto-proxying is inappropriate or accidental proxying for another. By resonating in your home frequency, by being still through STOIM, you can often cancel out inappropriate proxying in a matter of three minutes.

Poor nonphysical boundaries can also be a cause of proxying by accident. In Chapter Seven, SOS Clearing, you can find techniques to clear your energy field of wayward energies and shore up your nonphysical boundaries.

Sometimes just saying your full name three times out loud is enough to stop the proxying. Alternatively, you can try a TOLPAKAN Healing Directive:

> *I now command that* **fill in your name** *no longer proxy for another, now and in the future, in the highest and best way, in all directions of time, with ease and grace, and that anything preventing this from happening be immediately healed and resolved. Thank you.*

The reason we don't use the word "I" and instead use "your name" is because when you are proxying, you are not you. You are someone else in that moment. And to make sure that we deliver the healing precisely, we use your name while saying the directive. Make sense?

I've worked with a number of clients who have had chronic problems that could be traced to frequent proxying for others. For other clients, the proxying was due to a *spirit attachment*. When the proxying is due to a spirit attachment, sometimes we can figure out who it is, based on the person's history. For example, a woman came to my office to interview me to understand what kind of natural healing work I did. Because she was brand new, I decided to start with basic two-person muscle testing, thinking it would be simple.

Much to my surprise, after checking her polarity, I discovered that she was proxying for someone. On a whim, I asked her if anyone close to her had died within the last year or two. She promptly replied, "Yes, my father." I decided to muscle test her father's name. I asked her to first say her own name, "My name is Betty Brown," and her arm went weak. When I asked her to say her father's name, "My name is John Brown," her arm was strong. In other words, she was her father, not herself, energetically speaking. Her energy body was processing the unfinished business of her late father.

With her permission, I did some additional muscle testing and determined that her father's disembodied spirit was attached to her vagina. Now this information was probably the last thing I would've wanted to share with a person brand new to my practice, but despite my hesitation, I revealed this information to her, expecting her to bolt out the door.

But interestingly, Betty wasn't freaked out. She was intrigued. You see, her father had died of prostate cancer, so it made complete sense to her why we would have found his ghost attachment in her vagina. After further Divine Muscle Testing and some TOLPAKAN Healing, we determined quickly what her father needed to cross over, directed the healing, and *POOF!* he was gone. Betty suddenly felt lighter.

In the example of Betty, she was auto-proxying for a deceased loved one without even realizing it. It's possible that, over time, this energy drain could have manifested illness in her body, specifically her reproductive system.

Why does that happen? Especially for highly sensitive people, it often happens because their energetic boundaries can be weak.

There are seven different kinds of boundaries I know of:

- Physical

- Mental
- Emotional
- Spiritual
- Energetic
- Dimensional
- Relational

Any of the above could be weak and could potentially cause auto-proxying. Highly sensitive people are at higher risk of proxying for others because of their gift of being able to feel other people's energy.

If your polarity is correct and you are not proxying for someone or something else, then you can move on to the next step in the Check phase, which is Permission.

PERMISSION

The third step is to check if you have permission to ask this question. This is optional—not everybody needs to ask permission. If you feel like this question might be emotionally charged for you, however, then it may be useful to ask if you have permission to know the Divine True answer to this question.

For example, if a client asks about their five-year-old child's soul mission, I may not have permission to extract the soul mission until the child reaches a certain age. However, most adults have permission to extract their soul mission from the *Soul Mission Matrix*, a process I teach in the next chapter.

Establish the responses for yes and no; next, establish you're not auto-proxying. Next, ask whether you have permission. I like to do it out loud:

> *Do I have permission to ask about* _____ *and*
> *get a Divinely True answer right now through Divine Muscle*
> *Testing?*

By the way, the more specific the question, the better quality the answer you will receive. For example, if you ask, "Am I going to die?" meaning, will your spirit leave your body and will your physical body die, the answer would invariably be yes. A more specific question would be whether your physical body was going to die within a certain period of time. However, for this question, because it most likely will be emotionally charged, you may not get permission to know the exact date and time of death, if it isn't for your highest and greatest good to know ahead of time.

If you feel some sort of emotional attachment to the outcome, you can ask your spirit team or guardian angels to help you test objectively before you ask the permission question. If you get a yes answer to the permission question, then you can proceed to the next step in Divine Muscle Testing.

At this point, you might be thinking: *There seem to be many steps in learning Divine Muscle Testing.* I hear you. Just know that when these steps become your default modus operandi, you can fly through them and get to your answers quickly. My intention is to allow you the best accuracy possible, which is why I'm going through all the steps in great detail.

PERSUASION

The next step, persuasion, is also optional. Check if there are any of what we call *persuasive* or *leading energies* that might cause an incorrect answer. Sometimes I check for this if it's a very emotionally charged issue for the client, or the client feels that there's interference from others, whether they are humans, nonhumans, negative spirits, or they've had weak boundaries in the past.

Using the Body Sway method, ask:

> *Is it true that there are leading energies that will cause an untrue or incorrect answer through muscle testing right now?*

Alternatively, instead of asking a question, you can use a *statement* (something we'll review more of in the Predetermination step):

> *There are leading energies causing an incorrect or untrue answer through muscle testing right now.*

For some reason, we are able to catch more subtle leading energies using this type of question or statement than just a simple yes/no question.

For folks who are well practiced in muscle testing, you can be even more precise in catching super-subtle leading energies by doing the TOLPAKAN Countdown Method. If you get a no, that your testing is not being influenced by leading energies, you can challenge that by asking the following question:

> *How many leading energies are there causing an incorrect or untrue answer through muscle testing right now?*

Start with the number 10 and work your way down to a 0, muscle testing each answer until you get a yes response from your body. I can do this quickly, using a single-hand muscle testing method. From time to time, I'll catch a handful of leading energies. Once caught, I can usually just move into STOIM and do a TOLPAKAN Healing Directive to banish them and prevent them from interfering with my muscle testing. I'll share more about this in the Clearing phase of Divine Muscle Testing.

PREDETERMINATION

At the Predetermination step of the Check phase of Divine Muscle Testing, you are ensuring your questions are clear.

Some people feel strongly that one shouldn't ask questions, but instead offer statements. In my experience, both are fine, as long as you are very specific and clear about the information you are requesting. For example, you can ask:

Is eating a slice of organic whole wheat bread for my highest and greatest good today?

or you can state:

> *Eating a slice of organic whole wheat bread is for my highest and greatest good today.*

You should get the same response for both.

When testing food choices, I've noticed that some foods are neither "good" nor "bad" for us. In the above example, if you got a no, eating the slice of bread wasn't for your highest good, you may wish to query further, such as:

> *Is eating organic whole wheat bread harmful in any way to my body?*

You may also get a no. In that case you may ask:

> *Is eating organic whole wheat bread neutral for me? In other words, it is neither good nor bad for me. Is that true?*

Normally I don't like asking two questions in the same breath before getting an answer, but in this case, since both questions are directly related, I find it works for me.

As mentioned before, the specificity of the question is important, so I'd like to give you more examples of food-related questions you may wish to practice with. Say your goal is to lose excess belly fat, but you really enjoy eating bread and you think that's adding to the fat. You can muscle test how much bread you can eat that is safe or is for your highest good. For most humans, unless they have transcended and rewired much of their human programming and live in a state of constant joy and consciousness, the insulin spike from consuming two slices of organic whole wheat bread would be similar to eating a candy bar and would promote fat storage rather than fat burning.

The quality question you'd ask is:

> *Would eating a slice of organic whole wheat bread today be fully aligned with my goal of releasing excess body fat?*

Alternatively, you can ask a quality question that requires more muscle testing familiarity:

> *How many slices of organic whole wheat bread can I eat per week that would not interfere with my ability to release excess body fat as efficiently as possible? One? Two? Three?*

And so on. You would muscle test each number until you got a yes.

Experiment with both questions and statements, and find out what format works best for you. Feel free to share your experience with my private online community group. The link is in the Next Steps chapter. If you need help, tag me and I'll help you formulate your question or statement.

PHASE 3: CLEARING (OPTIONAL)

Before you start testing the actual questions, you can do an optional *Clearing* of leading energies. The TOLPAKAN Healing Directive you can use is:

It is commanded that all leading and hidden leading energies from any source, including personal biases and attachments, be cleared and released in the highest and best way, in all directions of time, in all realities where I exist. Thank you.

When I was learning, and I did not first ask permission if I was allowed to know the Divine True answer, I received nonsensical, unlikely answers. When this happened, I found a single leading energy that wasn't from personal or subconscious biases, mass consciousness, entities, or extraterrestrial interference. It was from Divine Source! In other words, I wasn't allowed to know the complete answer at that time. Because I didn't ask if I was permitted to know, Source diverted me so I would know I wasn't going to get a true answer.

In some rare instances, even the Universe will veer you away from the right answer because you're not really supposed to ask the question. You don't have permission to know at this time. This has happened to me only when I've been doing pretty heavy-duty healing with the assistance of my TOLPAKAN™ (TKH) Healing Method Guides 1, 2, and 3, which are included as part of the TOLPAKAN Healing Method Level 1 Training. This is a training program in my energy-healing Light Medicine modality. I've placed a link in the last chapter of this book if you'd like to learn more and watch a recording of a professional session with me and a volunteer.

For the most part, you don't have to worry about experiencing leading energies from Divine Source if you've already asked permission.

After doing the TOLPAKAN Clearing Directive, recheck to see if you have any other leading energies. If the answer is zero, you can ask your question and collect the answers.

PHASE 4: COLLECT

In the **Collect** phase, there are three steps: Stillness, Surrender, and Sense.

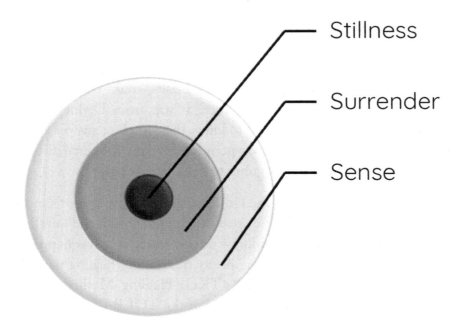

1. Go into *Stillness* (STOIM) to still the mind and get into the body.

2. *Surrender* to the answer, letting go.

3. Sense the answer in the body.

First, reconnect to Stillness. Go into STOIM. Feel the energy movement in your body. In that space, ask your question or say your statement out loud.

Next, surrender to the answer by simply letting go and being open to the answer coming through your body. If you stay in Stillness, you won't really have a problem here.

Lastly, sense what happens to your body after you ask the question and surrender to the answer. At the beginning, when you first try muscle testing, it might take up to three seconds for your body to respond with a yes or a no. As long as you've done all of your preparation ahead of time—connecting, checking, clearing (optional), and now collecting your answers—you'll find with frequent, fun practice, your body will respond faster and faster.

The two main reasons people do not succeed in Divine Muscle Testing is a lack of willingness to practice and a belief they can't do it. Like I said before, most children learn the technique lightning-fast. If a five-year-old can do it, you can do it too.

ADDITIONAL MUSCLE-TESTING TIPS

It's always a great idea to hydrate before a muscle-testing session. Drink eight to sixteen ounces of pure water beforehand. You can also activate the energy in your body, such as dancing around or doing the cross-crawl exercise twenty times.

If you're receiving confusing answers, remember to ask about whether you're allowed to get a Divinely True answer through muscle testing now.

If, even after much practice, you feel like your muscle testing is being interfered with because of wayward energies you cannot control, perform the additional clearing protocols in Chapter 7. Then, try again.

I have known of a few clairsentient students who aren't allowed to get their answers through muscle testing for various reasons. Most are being challenged to find their answers through an internal feeling in their body instead of an external movement of their body. Sometimes the feeling can be an emotion or an internal movement. I call this *Internal Muscle Testing*. It is a way to pay attention to the direction and quality of flow in STOIM and be able to discern a distinctive yes and no response.

One of the things I can do is to Divine Muscle Test at a distance without touching the other person. I teach my TOLPAKAN Healing Practitioner Trainees how to do this.

If you need help or guidance with your muscle testing or with asking quality questions, please post in our tribe's Light Warrior Network private online community, and remember to tag me by typing out my name.

Now that you've been taught Divine Muscle Testing, step-by-step, here is a summary of all the steps:

PHASE 1: CONNECT

- *Preparation* – of the body

- *Intention* – to connect to Source through STOIM

- *Direction* – say the TOLPAKAN Healing Directive

- *Attention* – to the body

PHASE 2: CHECK

- *Polarity* – are you balanced?

- *Proxy* – are you *you*?

- *Permission* – are you allowed to know the answer?

- *Persuasion* – are there leading energies?

- *Predetermination* – are the questions or statements you're testing clear?

PHASE 3: CLEAR (OPTIONAL)

Do the TOLPAKAN Clearing Directive to clear any wayward leading energies.

PHASE 4: COLLECT

- *Stillness* – get your mind still by focusing internally

- *Surrender* – let go of attachments and be open to the answers

- *Sense* – sense your body movement to see whether the answer is yes or no

Chapter Summary

1. Divine Muscle Testing is a great way to access your intuition through aligning with Divine Truth.

2. The Body Sway method is the easiest muscle-testing method to learn, whereby a sway forward is a yes response and a sway backward is a no response.

3. Being in Stillness (STOIM) optimizes your accuracy in muscle testing.

4. Divine Muscle Testing requires practice to become faster and more confident.

5. The quality of the question or statement you test determines the quality of the answer or information you receive.

6. Divine Muscle Testing and the TKH Guides 1, 2, and 3 are the foundational tools we use in the TOLPAKAN Healing Method to discover what's needed for optimal healing.

7. Internal Muscle Testing is a Divine Muscle Testing method that does not require outer movement of the body but relies on the perception of energy movement within the body.

Chapter 6

Soul Mission Matrix

THE REAL REASON YOU ARE HERE

After people have their daily physical needs taken care of—meaning a roof over their heads, clothes to wear, and food to eat—there comes a time when they ask themselves: *Why am I here?*

Many studies have confirmed the importance of a sense of purpose. Patrick Hill and Nicholas Turiano questioned more than 6000 people in a study about purpose and positive and negative emotions. People who reported a greater sense of purpose and direction in life were more likely to outlive their peers. Not only that, they had a 15 percent lower risk of death compared with those who said they were more or less "aimless." The cool thing is that it didn't seem to matter at what age the person found their direction, whether it was in their twenties, fifties, or seventies.

Have you ever wondered: *Why am I here?* or *What's my purpose?*

Probably every person you know has, on some level, wondered this about themselves. Without a purpose, humans seem to feel like something is missing from their lives. It is natural to believe life has meaning and is not random, even though outdated science may have told you when you were growing up that it was. Newer science has revealed that nature is not random. If you examine the structure of a seashell conch, a fiddlehead fern, or the cochlea of a human ear, you'll find that within them, and nearly all natural structures, is a mathematical formula called the *Golden Ratio*. The proportions of nature follow this pattern, and it is definitely not random.

Dolores Cannon was a well-known hypnotherapist who was particularly adept at extracting past-life information from her students and clients. After thousands upon thousands of readings, Dolores wrote in her book, *Three Waves of Volunteers*, about how her past-life readings started to morph and change. Under deep hypnotic regression, Dolores' subjects began sharing strange new insights about their past lives, including experiences as an alien on a spaceship or coming from a collective of pure "light" beings without a physical body. Prior to that, she mainly heard them describing past lives during points in history that were easily identifiable—a soldier in World War I, a priestess in ancient Egypt, or a healer who was burned at the stake in Salem because she was thought to be a witch.

Dolores revealed that when she asked these subjects under hypnosis why they were on this planet as a human, they would answer in one of three ways: Some said that they were here to resonate a certain vibration, such as Universal Unconditional Love. Dolores called that a *Being Mission*. Others said they had a job to perform, such as dismantling or revolutionizing our greed-driven, planet-killing ways. Think about the Occupy Wall Street movement, or the #metoo movement. She called this a *Doing Mission*. Yet others had both a Being and a Doing Mission here on Earth.

This pattern became so consistent that Dolores realized these souls were revealing something she was supposed to share with the rest of the world—these Sensitive Souls were volunteers who incarnated as humans to elevate the consciousness of humanity and save our planet.

According to Dolores, there are three waves of these volunteers: People in the first wave have a tough job. They are often the doers, the movers, and the shakers. There aren't too many people like them. They buck the system. They are revolutionaries and are often ostracized by their peers as being radical and too different. They are nonconformists, questioning why we do things the way we do. They reveal the inadequacies of our systems, and many are whistleblowers and shit-disturbers. Elizabeth Cady Stanton and other suffragettes, Mahatma Gandhi, Martin Luther King Jr., Rosa Parks, John F. Kennedy, and Gene Roddenberry (creator of *Star Trek*) are examples.

Some use their intuition and ingenuity to forever change the way we view and function in the world. They say yes to new ideas and possibilities when others say, "No, it can't be done." Nikola Tesla, Buckminster Fuller, Steve Jobs, Steven Spielberg, Marianne Williamson, and Brené Brown come to mind. There are so many more—many who live among us, who are not famous, who have made a difference just by being themselves. Maybe you are one of these first wave of volunteers. In spiritual circles, they are often called the *Indigos*.

The second wave of volunteers often have both Being and Doing Missions. These are our Generation X, Millennials, and Gen Z folks who are changing the landscape of commerce. Many are no longer buying brand names clothes to show off, for example, but are instead using their buying power to support companies with a heart and soul. For example, when I was looking for a pair of rainboots, I bought from a company that accepted its used boots back for recycling when they are no longer wearable. Rather than support giant agribusiness and factory-farmed meat, I buy meat and produce from the local farmers' markets. I can get toxin-free food and support my local farmers, even if I end up paying much more than at the grocery store.

The first two waves made way for the third wave of volunteers, who are the youngest. Most are babies and children as of this writing. According to Dolores, they have Being missions. They are gentler and softer in nature than the first wave folks and are here to anchor the vibration of love and peace. You can recognize these as babies who rarely cry, are almost always happy, and seem to be at peace, no matter what drama is going on around them. Being in their presence is like receiving an energy healing of love.

Not every volunteer or Sensitive Soul is an alien soul in human skin (also known as a *Starseed* or *Starperson*). I've met many who are angels. I know it might seem far-fetched, talking about aliens and all, but real, bona fide scientists have discovered billions of Earth-like planets rotating around a sun in our universe.[13] It would seem almost egotistical to think that we humans would be the only highly intelligent species around. Preposterous, actually. And as for angels, you only have to read books like Keith Leon S.'s, *Walking With My Angels* (Beyond Belief Books, 2019), to appreciate just how real angels are. Some of us are Earth angels. You might be one too.

Figuring out your Soul Type—Indigo, Angelic, or Starperson—is beyond what we can cover in this book, but it is something I teach in my TOLPAKAN Healing Method Level 1 Training. For more information on this program, please see the link in the Next Steps chapter. The good news is we can get you started on determining your Soul Mission using what I call the *Soul Mission Matrix*.

The three steps to determining your foundational Soul Mission in this lifetime are shown below:

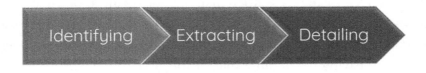

Identifying   Extracting   Detailing

13 Kunimoto, Michelle, and Jaymie M. Matthews. "Searching the Entirety of Kepler Data. II. Occurrence Rate Estimates for FGK Stars." *The Astronomical Journal.* 4 May 2020. DOI: 10.3847/1538-3881/ab88b0

STEP 1: IDENTIFYING

You'll be using Divine Muscle Testing, so follow the steps in Chapter Five to ready your mind, body, and spirit to receive Divine answers. Once you've connected to Stillness and are consistently receiving yes and no answers, then ask whether you have a Being Mission, a Doing Mission, or both in this lifetime:

- *Is my foundational Soul Mission in this lifetime a Being Mission right now?*

- *Is my foundational Soul Mission in this lifetime a Doing Mission right now?*

- *Is my foundational Soul Mission in this lifetime both a Being and a Doing Mission right now?*

The reason we ask "in this lifetime" is because we've had a small number of people test that they had more than one Being or Doing Mission, and from further questioning, I determined that certain missions from their other lives had been read by accident and that they weren't relevant to the current timeline. I know it sounds complicated, multiple lives and such, and beyond what we can cover in this book. Just know that if this subject interests you, you can learn more by studying some of my online programs, YouTube videos, or the Alternate Self Syndrome chapter I wrote for the bestselling book, *Evolutionary Healer*.

Once you've completed this step, write down your answers.

STEP 2: EXTRACTING

Using the Soul Mission Matrix below, use the first column if you have a Being Mission.

1. With Divine Muscle Testing, ask: *Is my Being Mission in this lifetime _____ ?* (fill in the blank with the first answer in the matrix)

2. If the answer is no, continue asking for each item going down the column until you get a solid yes.

Write down your answer.

If you have a Doing Mission:

1. Ask: *Is my Doing Mission in this lifetime* _____*?* (fill in the blank with the first answer in the matrix)

2. If the answer is no, continue asking for each item down the column until you get a solid yes.

Write down your answer.

Although there may be nuances to the type of Being and Doing Missions possible, the words in the Soul Mission Matrix seem to cover almost all the foundational missions we've discovered so far. Nevertheless, by being in Stillness, a different word might pop up in your awareness, so feel free to muscle test that possibility if it comes up.

THE SOUL MISSION MATRIX

BEING Mission	DOING Mission	DETAILS
Joy	Healing	WHO: humans, ETs, Indigos, women, men, children, spirits, animal, Mother Earth, all beings, galaxies, Earth angels?
Peace	Empowering	
Love	Grounding	
Acceptance	Integrating	
Oneness	Protecting	
Contentment	Teaching	WHAT: what is the format or process? 1-on-1, groups (how big?), etc.
Power	Counseling	
Awareness	Coaching	
Connection	Supporting	WHERE: location, geography
Openness	Innovating	
Compassion	Creating	WHEN: timeline; how soon?
Other	Transmuting	
	Transforming	WHY: higher purpose?
	Learning	
	Awakening	HOW: job? own business? free? for money?
	Communicating	
	Facilitating	
	Other	

STEP 3: DETAILING

In the third column, you'll see the words *Who, What, When, Where, Why,* and *How.* If you have solely a Being Mission, you need to focus only on Who. In other words, you're asking the Divine whom you are serving or helping in this timeline.

If you have a Doing Mission, you may be able to extract more details about your mission. Below I've outlined the kinds of questions you can ask to get yes/no answers from your Divine Muscle Testing:

Whom am I serving in this timeline?

- My family?

- My culture? (human)

- My collective? (star people)

- My country?

- Men? Women? Children?

- All of humanity? Living only? Deceased (no longer embodied)?

- All living beings?

- Mother Earth? Animals? Plants? Microbes?

- Other Sensitive Souls? (Indigos, Earth angels, Starseeds)

- The Cosmos (solar system, galaxy, Universe)

- Other: _____

(If you are new to my work, some of these may seem a little strange to you, but I've witnessed all sorts of missions when I've done this with my students and clients. Almost all people I've worked with have resonated with the answers extracted, even when I have not known the client well. If you get a no for everything on this list, go into Stillness and see if another word or picture pops into your mind. You can then confirm the answer with Divine Muscle Testing.)

What's the best format for me to express this mission?

- Working one-on-one with people?

- Working in groups?

- Working both one-on-one and groups?

- How large a group would be ideal to start with? Between one and fifty? Between fifty and one hundred?

(Keep muscle testing progressively narrower ranges: move to ranges of ten from here, then ask about specific numbers.) For some people the answer is "no limit."

- Am I doing this in person? In workshops? As a speaker? On podcasts?

- Am I doing this online? Remotely?

- Am I writing books? Blogs?

- Other: _____

Where is the best place for me to express my mission?

- Anywhere?

- A specific geographical location? Northern hemisphere? Southern hemisphere?

Keep asking for progressively smaller regions (i.e., from continent to country to province or state to city or town) until you narrow down the locale. The result will likely make sense to you, and you might have been already thinking of a particular location, even before determining your Soul Mission. You may want or need to move to a different location to express your mission. Every geographical location has its own energy signature. Some may be more beneficial to you than others. Hawaii, for example, is known in some spiritual traditions as the Heart Chakra of the planet. Many people feel at home when they first visit Hawaii, regardless of their cultural heritage or where they grew up. I felt that way in Waikiki despite the hustle and bustle of tourists shopping at high-end stores, something that I would normally try to stay away from.

When is the optimal time for me to express my mission?

- Now?

- Between now and six months from now?

- Between six months and a year from now?

- Beyond a year from now?

(Continue narrowing down the options by testing different time frames. For many adults, their mission will have started prior to the testing. You might get "now" as your answer. Sometimes you must wait because other things have to be in place for you to start your mission. That may mean a move, a divorce, or an ending of some sort.

Sometimes knowing your Doing Mission may be scary because if you've been ignoring those subtle inner signals to do something extraordinary, you feel a tad guilty. Please be gentle with yourself. Any anxiety during your testing will lead to less accurate answers. Just know there is always NOW.

Your life begins again in this moment. And again. And again. In each moment, you can make a different choice. And no one, not even God or your guardian angels, will judge you for making one choice or another. They may assist you in aligning with your Divine Path, but they will not force you.)

Why is this mission important? Why am I doing this?

- To save lives?

- To elevate the light or love on the planet?

- To evolve humanity?

- To protect others from dark forces?

- To create new positive morphic fields (blueprints)?

- To reinforce positive morphic fields already created?

- Other: _____

(If it is none of the above, you can go into Stillness and ask for the answer to drop in. For the grand majority of Sensitive Souls, the answer is often one of creating, reinforcing, or anchoring in positive morphic fields or blueprints for the masses to tap for healing and evolution.)

How am I to accomplish my Soul Mission?

- Do I get paid in the process?

  o Through employment?

  o Through my own business?

  o Through a charitable organization?

- For free?

  o Volunteering?

  o Philanthropy?

- Is it through my own business? Through a partnership?

- Other: _____

(The most common answer I've received when I've done Soul Mission readings with my clients is that the client is to start their own business, including consulting, teaching, coaching, training, and/or healing. It seems that Sensitive Souls gravitate to service businesses as compared to product businesses. That being said, some may end up selling or innovating health, wellness, or spiritual products. Commonly, when I do a reading on a client and find out that they ought to run their own businesses, they report they've been thinking of doing exactly that. These synchronicities are a way in which The Universe gives us confirmation of our own intuitive nudging, as subtle as it can be sometimes.)

Once you've written down your answers, congratulations are in order! Take some time to reflect on your answers and determine whether they truly resonate with you. Maybe walk away from it for a few days, and then come back to it with new eyes. See if your perspective changes.

After identifying, extracting, and detailing your foundational Soul Mission or Purpose for this lifetime, then it's time to own it.

Some students and clients who have done this process with me were expecting to discover their specific job title—artist, healer, and so on. Here's the thing: The Soul Mission Matrix helps determine your foundational mission *right now*. That doesn't mean that you can't express yourself in whatever capacity you wish for fun and exploration. As long as it is aligned to your foundational Soul Mission, you're good to go.

For example, if you've been thinking about producing and selling spiritual artwork online and your Soul Mission is a Being Mission of Love, it doesn't mean you shouldn't sell art. It just means that no matter what you choose to do, as long as you are resonating the morphic field or frequency of unconditional love, you're fulfilling your purpose. Similarly, if you have a Doing Mission of protecting Mother Earth, it doesn't mean you can't also start a local garden club, teaching children the value of growing food and flowers. Freely express yourself in any way you like because when you are healthy, happy, and prosperous, you will naturally give back and impact more people in a positive way.

Your Soul Mission doesn't have to take your whole lifetime. I've met many Sensitives who, because of their commitment to spiritual growth and evolution, have completed one mission and are on a new mission.

Furthermore, you can accept what I call *mini-missions* underneath the umbrella of your foundational Soul Mission. These mini-missions tend to be very specific and short-lived, but you are uniquely qualified to complete these jobs. For example, the TOLPAKAN Healing Method (TKH) healing frequencies are particularly good at healing dark energies, such as negative entities. From time to time, I'm called to heal entities infecting specific groups of beings that may intend to harm others. I'll usually get some sort of signal, either a symptom in my body, which is less preferred, or a curious electronic glitch in the electronic devices around me, which is more preferred; it usually means angels are trying to get my attention.

Using TKH and a very rapid succession of quality questions, I can quickly determine the cause of the issue and heal it on a small or large scale, depending on the need, and then return to going about my business.

Once you've determined your Soul Mission, feel free to post it in my private online community for Sensitive Souls. Remember to tag me so I can celebrate with you.

Chapter Summary

1. Many Sensitive Souls are here to serve others and are volunteers to help raise the consciousness and vibration of the planet.

2. Your foundational Soul Mission/Purpose can be determined using a three-step process and the Soul Mission Matrix.

3. If you feel you have completed your Soul Mission, you can return to the three-step process to find your next Soul Mission.

4. Mini-missions are shorter, smaller missions under the umbrella of your bigger, foundational Soul Mission.

Chapter 7

SOS Clearing

FEEL CLEAR. FEEL FREE

Next, I show you ways of clearing negative energy from your energy field so you can feel clearer, calmer, and more confident. My students have noted that clearing their energy fields regularly has helped them feel more energized and more rested. They also feel like they are in a better mood and sleep better at night.

Because you have already learned Stillness thought STOIM, you already have a fantastic way of auto-clearing energies that aren't yours. Yes! By practicing Stillness, you are immersed in your own energy. Anything that isn't you easily dissipates. In this chapter, you will learn several additional ways to clear negative energy, as well as how to minimize your reactivity to negative energy. Cool?

If I start to feel irritable or upset, seemingly for no reason, one of two things happens. If I don't catch it soon enough, I create a logical reason why I'm irritable, pinning the blame on people around me. If I do catch it in time, then the first question I ask is: *Whose stuff is this?* This one question alone has changed my life immeasurably.

Using Divine Muscle Testing, I can quickly figure out if what I'm feeling is mine or someone else's. At times, the irritability I feel is simply my sensitivity Superpowers of empathy on overdrive. It happens to every highly sensitive person from time to time, especially during the ascension process. We suddenly *feel too much*. Knowing what to do in these circumstances is the name of the game and can mean the difference between our sensitivity being a nightmare or a gift. The *ascension process* is what spiritual leaders refer to when they talk about the naturally occurring rise of spiritual energy in the cosmos. It's a good thing. But for Sensitive Souls, it can expand our sensitivity gifts multifold, and that can be uncomfortable if we don't know how to rein them in.

Sometimes, because I have certain responsibilities based on my soul mission, it is for my highest and greatest good to feel *negative stuff*, at least temporarily. It allows me to know what's going on in the world, and I can clear it for everyone. For example, I often know if there is a psychic attack on the collective unconscious. Something big like that can affect millions, so I get to know about it before it does real damage, and I can easily clear it.

Most people do not carry that level of spiritual responsibility to heal mass consciousness or Mother Earth or something bigger than themselves, but I'm sharing that information in case you are one of them. Muscle testing using the Soul Mission Matrix, found in Chapter 6, will give you some idea.

For the most part, knowing how to clear yourself is essential. It's a skill I think everybody—especially highly sensitive people—should know. I would love for highly sensitive parents to teach it to their children as well.

Now let's go over some science related to negative energy. In one fascinating study,[14] scientists took gamma-irradiated cells, (genetically

---

14 Jones, Joie P. and Yury Kronn. "New Understandings on the Effects of Energetic Pollution on the Healing Process and Solutions Made Possible with Modern Subtle Energy Technology." *Medical Week, Baden-Baden.* October 2008; Jones, Joie P. "An Extensive Laboratory Study of Pranic Healing Using Contemporary Medical Imaging and Laboratory Methods." *Irvine Invited Presentation for the Seventh World Pranic Healers' Convention,* Mumbai, India, May 12–14, 2006. equilibrium-e3.com/images/PDF/Jones%20Pranic%20Healing%20

identical cells in petri dishes that were purposefully damaged), and exposed them to three different lab environments and measured their rate of healing.

In the *conditioned lab*, pranic healers "cleaned" the lab by removing "dirty energy" and "energizing with positive energy." This "cleaning" process took four months before the healers felt that the lab was sufficiently "clean" to undertake the experiments. The *non-conditioned lab* was a fairly new and well-maintained environment. The dirty lab was a lab where experiments on dissected animals and other similar experimentation had been conducted over a lengthy period of time.

The gamma-irradiated cells were placed in each of the three labs. Pranic healers sent energy healing to all the cells over a period of time. The cells that were placed in the conditioned lab had an impressive 88 percent survival rate. The cells in the non-conditioned lab had a 10 percent survival rate, and the cells in the dirty lab had a 0 percent survival rate. This study dramatically illustrates how dirty energy can affect living systems.

Think about it. If you have an argument in the home or you're watching a horror movie or the news, negative energy has been deposited in your space. If a chronically depressed friend visits you every day complaining about how miserable their life is, they leave traces of low vibrational energy in your space. It infects the space and, therefore, has the potential to infect you and your energy field.

We regularly bathe our bodies, brush our teeth, and shampoo our hair. Why? What would happen if we did not do those things? We would get dirty and smelly, and no one would want to be around us, right? The same is true of your energy field.

Research.pdf

Many of us take our energy fields for granted because most of us can't see them with the naked eye. We don't even know an energy field is there. Instead of cleaning and taking care of it, we ignore it, and it becomes super, super dirty. Then we wonder why we don't feel good, 'cause guess what? Our energy fields are connected to our bodies and all of our organs. There is an interaction between the energy of the organs and our energy fields and vice versa.

If your energy field is dirty and unhappy and filled with low, negative energy, eventually this will affect your physical, mental, and emotional health.

There are few of us who are sufficiently robust and flexible in our energy fields that we can withstand—with ease—a never-ending onslaught of negative vibes in our own home. You may have already experienced the energy-draining effects of it in your life. It is crucial for all of us to learn how to clear our energetic fields regularly. That doesn't mean that you shouldn't take real-world actions to improve your home situation. I'm not talking about evicting your sick and dying grandmother. I'm talking about having healthy boundaries and not letting people use or abuse you in any way.

In this chapter, you can learn multiple energy healing techniques to clear your energy field. You can check and test each one to see which one works best for you. They are presented in no particular order, but I suggest you try each of them and see how you feel afterward. Done regularly, you can sense an incredible shift afterward in the health of your energy field and how you feel physically, emotionally, and mentally.

Before we discuss the techniques, let's talk about the kinds of negative vibrations you can have in your energy field. We don't have room in this chapter to name all of them, but some of the common causes include negative emotions and thoughts from yourself or other people.

Negative spiritual energies can enter your space as well. Different energetic toxins, including electromagnetic radiation, can also be present.

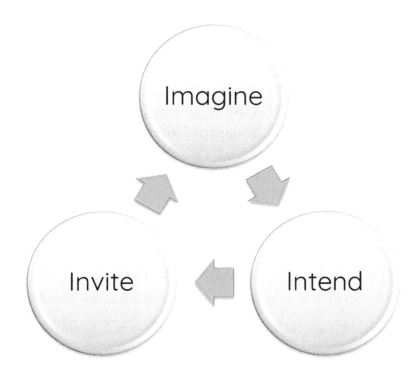

There are three steps to the clearing process, and that's true for all of the processes we cover in this chapter.

1. *Imagine* the ideal outcome or results.
2. *Intend* the clearing or healing.
3. *Invite* in positive energy and support.

ASTRAL CONNECTION CONTROL

Your astral connection is an opening of your crown that allows you to access higher states of consciousness and other dimensions when you are in a meditative state or a state of love or peace.

The astral connection helps you connect, receive, and see. One of the teachers who helped me connect with my gifts to transmute dark energies is healer Tamara Joy Patterson. Tamara says:

When [astral connection] is too open too often, and the person is in a lower vibrational state, this opening can allow excess psychic information, attack, and so on, to "haunt" the person. If it is too open in an unhealthy way, it can be exacerbated by a lack of being able to root for the reasons of HPA overstimulation due to the subconscious beliefs: I am unsafe or I am unsupported. In clients (who) are sick (and) need to be in their body and heal, I ask for it to close. In moderately awake and healthy clients, I recommend that it be balanced, and we test it throughout the day.[15]

I used to start skating at the rink, only to realize I was discombobulated and wasn't centering my spins. After a number of occasions, I realized that if I balanced my astral connection before stepping out onto the ice, I was able to center my spins and skate in a more grounded manner.

For people who are feeling or sensing way too much, this is a great strategy: Close and/or balance your astral connection. It's a simple procedure. Now, if you do Divine Muscle Testing, you can check how open your astral connection is. Ask "How balanced is my astral connection?" and then test for a response to numbers along a scale from 0 to 100 percent.

Many highly sensitive people's astral connections are wide open. Now, is that a problem? Well, in some cases it is. When doing healing work, often we connect to higher realms of consciousness because it's necessary to access information for our clients. However, if a we are not grounded or rooted properly, this can cause some problems, particularly burnout.

---

15 Personal email correspondence

It's necessary to manage that astral connection. Using Divine Muscle Testing, you can investigate by asking: "How open should my astral connection be for my highest and greatest good while I'm at home? When I'm at the shopping mall? When I'm at the arena watching a hockey game?" and ask for a percentage. The number can vary among people. Some people who have experimented with hallucinogenic drugs, for example, may have their astral connections burst wide open, whereby it is dangerous or unhealthy for them. We have to teach them how to close it or manage it.

CLOSING THE CONNECTION

Not everybody wants to learn to muscle test, so I have developed a TOLPAKAN Healing Directive that helps you balance and close your astral connection.

Step 1: *Imagine* your astral connection as a cone-shaped area of light above your head. You may be able to sense how open it is by sending your attention to this area. Put your hand on top of your head, and imagine this cone becoming narrower.

Step 2: With the *intention* of managing and balancing, say this directive out loud:

> *I now command that my astral connection be closed and balanced in the highest and best way, and that it become so whenever it's for my highest and greatest good. Thank you.*

Step 3: *Invite* your guardian angels and spirit support team to help you manage your astral connection at all times and remind you to close it when it is for your highest good.

If you've asked for it to close and it's not for your highest and greatest good to completely close, it won't close. For most people, it will stay open only a small percentage. You don't have to worry about it closing down completely. If you're moderately healthy, your astral connection may be more open because you're able to handle that amount of information without being susceptible to psychic attacks. If you're more grounded, you're more rooted, you're more embodied, and you're not totally stressed out all the time, then, your astral connection may remain fairly open and still test as being 100 percent balanced.

My astral connection tends to be very open, now that I can handle a lot of psychic information without being overwhelmed by it. I have good boundaries and excellent discernment. Sometimes I ask for the connection to close, and it doesn't because it isn't for my highest good.

Let's review. If you do Divine Muscle Testing, you can check two different things if you wish. You can check how open your astral connection is currently and how open it should be for the highest good, or you can check how *balanced* it is currently out of 100 percent—not concerning yourself with exactly how open it is and what would be the ideal percentage for you. After completing the three steps above (imagine, intend, invite) to balance and close your astral connection, you can, if you wish, recheck your answers.

If a sensitive person plans to venture into a public area with lots of people, I recommend closing the astral connection before they leave the house. That has the ability to profoundly reduce the stress of feeling too much, which means they can enjoy their outings with greater calm and peace.

GROUNDING

You may have heard of grounding before. There are many different types of grounding. There is electromagnetically grounding, in which you put your bare skin on the earth, and the negatively charged electrons from the Mother Earth come into your body and release inflammation. They balance the positively charged toxin particles in your body.

That's not the type of grounding we're talking about here. We're talking about spiritual grounding. Many people run around with their energy scattered all over the place. You may experience them as being flighty or having their head in the clouds.

Typical symptoms of not being spiritually grounded include:

- Being chronically ill

- Feeling spacey or *like an airhead*

- Being accident prone

- Having chronic unexplained dizziness

- Never having enough money

- Floating from one thing to another without accomplishing much

- Feeling directionless or changing directions so often that nothing tangible manifests

In order to heal the body, our energies need to *be* embodied—that is, be in the body. During sleep, your astral body (the spiritual version of your physical body) often travels outside the body. Many people who have documented near-death experiences have similar stories about floating above their physical bodies, being able to see and hear everything around them. The astral body is connected to the physical body through a cord called the *astral cord*. When someone dies, this cord is naturally severed and the spirit leaves the body permanently.

Being ungrounded is like waking up from sleep with your astral body not fully back into your physical body. Being ungrounded not only makes it difficult to physically heal, it makes it difficult to manifest anything tangible in the 3D world. You may have known gifted healers who have been grossly and dangerously overweight, barely made ends meet, or experienced repetitive traumatic events. These are all symptoms of having difficulty grounding.

Being grounded affords you the protection of having all your energies embodied. Being ungrounded is like living in a busy neighborhood and leaving your front door wide open for anyone to just waltz in and take over your house. Not good, especially when you come back home to find the place trashed and your jewelry missing.

Let's go over the three steps to become grounded.

Step 1: *Imagine* a big tube or cord the width of your energy field. If you outstretch your arms, this is the minimum width I want you to make it. This is something that I heard from my healer friend, Lottie Cooper. She advises making a grounding cord that is a lot bigger than most. Picture the cord coming out of the bottoms of the tailbone and feet.

Step 2: *Intend* that anything that isn't 100 percent Divine love, light, and truth be sent down the grounding cord deep into the earth to be transmuted. Some people imagine, experience, or see darkness, dirt, or debris sucked down this humongous grounding cord.

Step 3: Once you feel you are done with grounding the stuff you don't need nor want, then it is time to *invite* positive, healing energies from Mother Earth to travel up the cord into your body and auric field, all the way up past the crown of your head, to connect you to both Heaven and Earth.

You can do this technique sitting or standing. Any negative energy draining out of you is transmuted by Mother Earth. Don't worry, she can handle it. That's what she does. She has her own set of spiritual helpers.

I recommend grounding every morning as you step out of bed and any time you feel spacey, confused, tired, or weak. As an extra bonus, if you do your grounding technique while your bare feet are exposed to the earth (that includes standing in a lake or ocean), you'll receive the added benefit of being electromagnetically grounded. That means that harmful, toxic EMF inflammatory energies are neutralized as the Earth's electrons travel up your body. Talking on the cell phone while you are standing barefoot on the grass is much safer than when you have shoes on.

THE WATERFALL MEDITATION

I'm a big fan of waterfalls. This is a fun and beautiful way of clearing and cleaning your energy field, and it's great to do in the shower in the morning or evening when you come home from work.

Step 1: *Imagine* what it feels like to be under a beautiful refreshing waterfall.

Step 2: Make the *intention* that all negative, low-vibrational energies are washing away from you, inside and out. Feel how clean it feels. All that negative energy is scrubbed and released from your auric field and body and becomes transmuted by Mother Earth.

Step 3: Lastly, *invite* positive energies from the water to charge your energy field with positive energy. Water is a carrier of information, so it is a wonderful conduit for positive energies to flow to you.

Pay attention to how you feel before and afterward. You'll have a new-found love for showers and waterfalls now.

ETHERIC CORD-CUTTING

We interact with various people every day, and those interactions create energetic cords between us. It is a natural phenomenon, so don't freak out! Simply thinking about a person can create a cord with that person. It's probably why, when someone comes to mind, they call you unexpectedly.

Part of this completely natural phenomenon is the dissolution or disappearance of the cords soon after your interaction with other people. For many of us, however, we attach to these cords. After a while, we look like Dr. Octopus from the Spider-Man comic book series, with cords attached to various parts of our bodies. Most energy healing experts feel that being *corded* to others is unhealthy, especially if you are dragging around a bunch of cords. Some believe that this can contribute to being overweight. Others believe that the cords can drain you of your energy, especially if you are corded to someone who is an *energy vampire*.

An energy vampire is a person who sucks energy from another to feed themselves. Most energy vampires don't know they are behaving this way, but you certainly do because you feel drained when you are around them. Dr. Judith Orloff explains the different types of energy vampires and how to deal with them in her book, *The Empath's Survival Guide: Life Strategies for Sensitive People.* She talks about energy vampire personalities, such as the Narcissist, The Rage-aholic, The Drama Queen, The Victim, and The Passive Aggressive.

In Dr. Bradley Nelson's *The Body Code,* heart-to-heart cords between people are considered normal and healthy and generally do not need to be removed. However, there may be many other types of cords that can drain your energy.

There are cords that are not the natural ones created by human-to-human interaction. We're not going to cover those in this book, but

I can tell you that some of these other cords are highly negative and put in place intentionally by low-vibrational spirits. Even if you don't know about these cords, you can cut them using your intention by following the three steps outlined below.

Step 1: *Imagine* your hands like lasers, or light sabers if you're a *Star Wars* fan. Start at the top of your body. Cut away any cords on your front, all the way down underneath each foot. Next, cut away cords down the back of you. You can imagine the lasers being lengthy enough so that you don't have to bend too far to cut the cords attached to your back or your lower body. Remember to cut the cords on both arms as well.

Step 2: While cutting these cords, you *intend* that these cords are cut and dissolved, sealing the ends (flush to your body) with Love. There's nothing violent or traumatic about it. It's very gentle and loving.

Step 3: *Invite* positive healing energies to automatically clean your aura of negative cords, now and in the future. In the TOLPAKAN Healing Method, you can set up a TKH Clearing Vortex inside your auric field to auto-clean negative energy. Once you've set it up, all you need to do is go into Stillness (STOIM) to reboot it.

The TKH Clearing Vortex is a positive morphic field that I have set up and co-created with the Universe to help you automatically clean your auric field of negative energy and negative cords. Whether this works 100 percent of the time for you depends on your level of spiritual responsibility. In other words, if you have to be more spiritual responsible than the average person because of your soul's evolution, then you may have to consciously do the etheric cord-cutting technique on a regular basis.

THE AURA SCRUBBER

The fourth SOS technique is called the *Aura Scrubber*. And by the way, we go over all of these SOS techniques in the live and in-person Light Warrior Training Camp. The camp is super-fun and you receive immediate feedback from me on how well you are doing with each technique. By the end of camp, when you re-enter the wider world, you'll carry an increased sense of confidence in your new skills.

Scrubbing the aura easily clears your aura of negative energy. It isn't better or worse than any of the other techniques I've shown you. I share a variety of techniques because some people gravitate more to one than another. The Aura Scrubber is a great one to teach young children because they have excellent imaginations.

Step 1: *Imagine* your hands beaming with light. These are your scrubbers. If you can imagine your aura as a sphere all around you, you're going to be on the inside just scrubbing away, clearing it of all sorts of negative energy. Sort of like in the movie, *The Karate Kid*: "wax on, wax off."

Step 2: Make the *intention* that your hands of light will know where to clear and clean all parts of your aura. Let your intuition direct your hands wherever they feel moved—move your scrubbers all around you to get every bit of your aura clean. Just wash, wash, wash. Make the intention to wash everything inside and out of your auric field. Not only is this fun—especially for kids—you get a bit of an upper body workout in the process.

Step 3: While scrubbing, *invite* positive energy to restore your boundaries, filling any holes that might be present in your auric field. Holes can occur for various reasons, including trauma, cords, or energy weapons piercing your energy field. Using this procedure, you can seal these holes so that your boundaries are sovereign. Try this technique and see how it feels compared to Grounding and the Waterfall Meditation.

TOLPAKAN CLEARING DIRECTIVE

In this last clearing technique, you say a TOLPAKAN Clearing Directive out loud. It is easy and might be your go-to clearing technique if you're in hurry. A TOLPAKAN (TKH) Directive is like a command to the Universe to create a new desired reality for you. They work most effectively when you can connect to Stillness, even for a few seconds, as you say the Directive. In the Directive, you'll notice the word *microbiome*. The microbiome referred to here is the community of trillions of cells of beneficial bacteria and other micro-organisms living in the human body. The reason I've added it into the Directive is that I have found that their health and well-being have a huge impact on yours, so we might as well heal "them" as we are healing "you."

Step 1: Get into Stillness (do STOIM). *Imagine* that your entire being is being cleansed, cleared, and filled with light and that this light emanates and expands to all universes to all versions of you.

Step 2: *Intend* for the clearing to affect you on all levels: physically, mentally, emotionally, spiritually, energetically, dimensionally, and relationally, and for it to be done with ease and grace. Say out loud:

> *I now command that all energies less than 100 percent aligned with Source love, light, and truth be cleared and dissolved and uncreated for me, all parts of me, including my energy field and my microbiome and all timelines where I exist, in the highest and best way with ease, speed, and grace. Thank you.*

Step 3: *Invite* your God team or angelic team of 100 percent love, light, and truth to support you at all times.

With just a little practice, you'll be able to complete this clearing in a matter of seconds. Your ability to be Still by first focusing on the movement inside your body, then imagining your desired outcome while you say the TKH Directive, will make you a powerful self-healer.

THE CLEARING AND PROTECTION SPRAY FORMULA

To use my Clearing and Protection Spray™ Formula, first watch the TOLPAKAN Healing energy-infused video. With your focused intention, you then charge—or infuse with positive healing energy—a container of water. I advise finding a clean spray bottle (like the colorful ones you see at housewares stores), filling it with clean water, and adding a pinch of Himalayan crystal salt to help hold the energy.

The Clearing and Protection Spray Formula is simple to use and is infused with a number of high-vibrational energies that help to clear negative energies, including ghosts, entity and ET portals, and dirty electromagnetic energies, while at the same time creating a protective shield in the room that lasts around twenty-four hours. To get my free Clearing and Protection Spray Formula, just go to clearingandprotectionspray.com to download it.

To charge your water, follow these three steps:

Step 1: *Imagine* the positive energies flowing into the water you are paying attention to, as you view the video.

Step 2: *Intend* for the positive energies to charge the water by just paying attention to the water, either by looking at it or seeing it in your mind's eye in case the bottle is in a different location.

Step 3: *Invite* the positive energies to be infused into the water.

Charge the water with these energies by playing the video and basically telling the energies infused in the video to charge a specific bottle of water. Although the video is three minutes long, only nine seconds or so are needed for the water to fully charge, and then you can use it. The charged water can be sprayed to clear energy, or drunk as an energy-clearing elixir. You can charge any body of water. The effects are only limited by your ability to focus your attention and imagination.

Spray your entire house one to two times per week and your bedroom every night before bed for more restful sleep. In rooms with a lot of electronic equipment, it may be wise to spray more often. Use a fine mist to avoid soaking your equipment with water. You can also spray yourself when you come home every day from work or school for a quick pick-me-up. It's a great way to leave the stresses of the day behind and feel more energized and awake when you greet your family. Remember to spray your car once in a while, too, especially if you've had other people in it.

When I travel, I often pack an empty spray bottle. I make up the Clearing Spray at my destination and spray the hotel room and entryway every day. It helps me sleep better, wake up refreshed, and feel calmer amid all the energy of people and EMF around me.

Please note that if you charge liquid you wish to drink, it will likely change the taste. Soda may taste less sugary or even seem flat. Wine or alcohol may taste less appealing, so be mindful of what you choose to charge with this formula.

Young children who are afraid of monsters in their room can be given their own spray bottle to decorate with stickers and bling. Parents and caregivers can help them fill it up with water and even add nice-smelling essential oils, such as lavender or grapefruit, and show the children how to charge the water by playing the video. Once the water is charged, children can use this spray to "heal the monsters" so that they can go to a better place where they will be happier. One three-year-old who did this not only got rid of the monster in his room, he got rid of an entity portal in the hallway. Another patient's sensitive child was seeing ghosts. They equipped the child with a Clearing Spray bottle next her bed so she could "spray the people" she would occasionally see at night when she woke up from sleep.

Chapter Summary

1. By clearing your energy field, you remove energies that can potentially cause moodiness, anxiety, and pain.

2. Energy clearing should be a daily habit, just like brushing your teeth or washing yourself, so you may feel freer, lighter, and more balanced.

3. Closing or balancing the astral connection is a great technique to prevent excessive psychic information for sensitive people who need to spend time in places with a lot of people.

4. Grounding, The Waterfall Meditation, and Aura Scrubbing are three different ways of clearing the energy field. Choose the one(s) that work best for you.

5. Etheric cord-cutting helps to remove unnecessary energy cords between you and another being. In doing so, you contain your energy and prevent excessive energy drain.

6. TOLPAKAN Healing Directives can be used to quickly clear all parts of yourself in multiple timelines at once. Begin by doing STOIM for greatest effect.

7. The Clearing and Protection Spray is a quick way to clear energy. You can teach children to use it, even for perceived threats such as monsters and ghosts.

SECTION 2

SENSING

Chapter 8

Transformational Telepathy

CONFLICT RESOLUTION MADE EASY

In this chapter, we focus on *Basic Transformational Telepathy,* a technique that you can use to quickly resolve conflict and harmonize relationships.

How many of you have had the experience of thinking about contacting a specific person, then that person calls, emails, or just plain shows up somewhere unexpectedly? Many have. Is that intuition, telepathy, or both?

In 2014, a study by an international team of researchers[16] discovered a noninvasive method to transmit conscious thought between one human brain and another. Telepathy is real and you can use it to your advantage.

Dr. Rupert Sheldrake has done fascinating research into telephone telepathy and animal telepathy. He said it "led me to see telepathy as a normal, rather than a paranormal phenomenon." His research is summarized in his 2003 book *The Sense of Being Stared At and Other Aspects of the Extended Mind.*[17]

---

16 Carles Grau et al. "Conscious brain-to-brain communication in humans using non-invasive technologies." *PloS One.* 2014; 9(8). DOI: 10.1371/journal.pone.0105225

17 Sheldrake, Rupert. *The Sense of Being Stared At And Other Aspects of The Extended Mind* (Hutchinson, London, 2003; Crown, New York, 2003). A fully revised and updated edition was published in the U.S. in 2013 (Inner Traditions, Rochester, VT). sheldrake.org/research/telepathy

"Fred," a former patient of mine, had fibromyalgia and chronic fatigue syndrome. He came into the office one day extremely agitated. His son had just tried to commit suicide. Fred had hardly slept since the news, and he was so upset that he was literally shaking. I felt bad for him, especially since he was not well himself.

Fred felt guilty for not being at his son's side in the hospital. He could barely take care of himself, let alone muster up the money and energy to fly across the country to be with his son. Given his condition, I asked Fred if he'd be willing to help his son from a distance.

"If there were something easy you could do that wouldn't cost you anything, but would make a huge positive impact on your son, would you be willing to do it for thirty days?"

Fred's answer was a resounding, "Yes!"

I taught Fred to do Transformational Telepathy, and he promised he would do it for thirty days in a row to help his son. I eagerly awaited Fred's return to my office so I could hear the results of his efforts.

Almost six weeks later, Fred finally came into the office. The first thing I asked him was, "How is your son?"

And he looked at me curiously and he said, "What about my son?"

I said, somewhat surprised, "Well, you know, the son who was hospitalized for attempting suicide?"

With eyes opening wide and a smile on his face, he said, "Oh! He's just great!" Apparently, his son miraculously got better, was no longer depressed or suicidal, and had been discharged from the hospital without needing any medications. He had returned to work full time.

Powerful stuff!

The spoken language, wonderful as it is, may not be the most efficient way to communicate. Bestselling author Dolores Cannon, author of *The Three Waves of Volunteers*, documents that many of the thousands of people she's performed hypnotic regressions for, in which the participants lived other lives as what we could call *extraterrestrials*— nonhuman beings from other planets—recounted being able to communicate without opening their mouths or making a sound. The communication was through telepathy, in which images and feelings are shared instead of words. Popular culture, interestingly, also demonstrates this ability in various sci-fi movies such as *Avatar*, the Harry Potter series, and *The Dark Crystal*. In ancient and indigenous cultures, shamans and spiritual leaders receive intuitive information telepathically from spiritual sources.

The skill of Transformational Telepathy is one in which you communicate with another person without spoken words. They receive this communication from you, even if they don't know you're sending it. The Basic Transformational Telepathic method is highly profound despite its simplicity. It is often used for smoothing over conflict between two people when a face-to-face confrontation may be volatile or incredibly uncomfortable. Basic Transformational Telepathy is especially effective when conflict is present, such as when you've had an argument with a loved one and you're not speaking to each other, or if you've had a misunderstanding with a friend and spiteful words were exchanged, or if your boss at work is giving you a hard time, and you are frustrated and angry.

You're probably curious about how Transformational Telepathy works. From a quantum physics perspective, and from an energy healer's perspective, every emotion or thought is a *quantum*, or packet, of light energy. In quantum physics, they are called *photons*. When you are feeling angry at someone, the other person can perceive this anger energy as something attacking or pushing against them. Whether you think you're hiding your feelings well or not, the other person still receives this packet of energy.

When someone perceives negative energy coming their way, their natural response is to resist it. It's like pushing against a wall that doesn't want to budge. Negative energy is wasted energy, and no one wins. When you use Transformational Telepathy, the conflictual energy is dissolved by love and appreciation. The other person receives a packet of appreciation energy, and there is no resistance coming from them. It's almost as if you're doing a mini-healing on them.

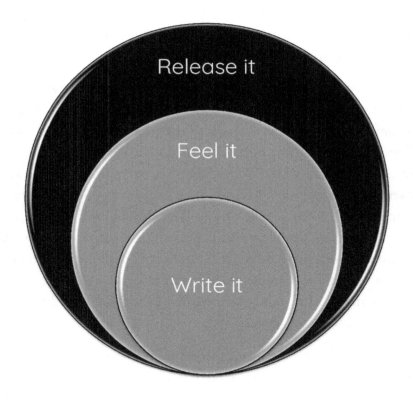

1. *Write it* – ten things you appreciate
2. *Feel it* – the appreciation
3. *Release it* – residual energies of resistance

Step 1: *Write It*. Using a blank piece of paper or a journal, write the name of a person you have a conflict with or with whom you'd like to have a better relationship. Include the date. List under their name ten things you appreciate about the person. I know it might not be easy to think of good things to say if you're upset with someone, but do the best you can. If you know this person well, then focus on their positive qualities—what they do well, even if it doesn't pertain to you personally. If you don't know them well, you may have to rewind in your mind what you *do* know about them and extrapolate the appreciation from what you've observed.

Examples include:

- *I appreciate you for making my coffee each morning.*
- *I appreciate you for being on time.*
- *I appreciate you for how you tend your garden.*
- *I appreciate you for loving animals.*
- *I appreciate you for your devotion to being a great single mom.*
- *I appreciate you for having the coolest-colored socks.*
- *I appreciate you for how neat and tidy you keep your desk.*
- *I appreciate you for being a great cook.*

Step 2: *Feel It*. Once you start actively looking for and writing down things what you appreciate about the person you have a conflict with, it becomes easier to feel the appreciation. Feel it in your body, not just your mind. What you focus on grows. Good feelings, when embodied, are natural healing remedies. Even if you are angry and upset about what they did to you, by appreciating their positive traits, your feelings follow your focus. While you write, consciously make the intention of feeling the feelings of appreciation, even if you're aware that you are resisting the exercise. It's okay. Do what you can. With practice you'll be amazed by how quickly your feelings just flow with your shift of focus.

I know, I know. You're probably thinking: *What if they are a narcissist, and I can't find any good traits?* In that case, appreciate their skills as a narcissist. Appreciate them for their ability to manipulate a situation to their favor, how skillfully they deflect blame onto others, or how charismatic they are while they're trying to manipulate you. You never know; in a hostage situation, those skills might come in handy! Be creative. Besides, if you are in a romantic relationship with a narcissist, remember that there must have been something you liked about this person; otherwise, you wouldn't be in a relationship with them.

Step 3: *Release it.* Once you've written your list (feel free to write more than ten things if you're in a groove), and you've felt the feelings of appreciation in your body, now release any residual resistance or anger you feel. Think of the residual resistance as energetic residue from the past. There are several ways to release this energy:

- You can use *Heart Tapping*, an energy-release technique, where you tap on your breast bone close to your heart center while making the intention to release it. Just one to three minutes of tapping is usually enough. Dr. John Diamond, in his book, *Life Energy*, has demonstrated that tapping the thymus gland, which is situated beneath your breast bone, can temporarily balance all your energy meridians—energy pathways described by Chinese Medicine thousands of years ago.[18] In addition to releasing energetic residue, you are doing something healthy for yourself.

- You can ask your Spirit Team, God Team, or guardian angels to help you release this excess unproductive energy. In my experience, they are more than happy to assist you in this process; however, they need your request to intervene because

18 Diamond, John. *Life Energy: Using the Meridians to Unlock the Hidden Power of Your Emotions.* Paragon House, 1990.

of the law of free will. When I'm having a moment and I need to vent, I go to the forest and talk to my angels. Once I've vented, I ask them to help me resolve the uncomfortable feelings I'm harboring. Normally it doesn't take long for those feelings to subside, and often, loving feelings take their place.

- You can also use the TOLPAKAN Healing Method to help you release negative energy. Go into STOIM and feel your body and its flow. Once you are there, use the TOLPAKAN Directive:

  I now command that all negative, low-vibrational, uncomfortable energy that I'm experiencing be released, dissolved, and uncreated in the highest and best way, in all directions of time, in all timelines where I exist, with ease and grace. Thank you!

  See how you feel a minute or two afterward.

It is highly recommended to do Basic Transformational Telepathy for thirty days straight to radically transform a relationship. If you have a troubled teen or family member, ongoing daily telepathy is incredibly healing for both parties. You'll be amazed at the difference in their behavior. You can address multiple people or relationships simultaneously.

Sometimes people ask me if they can reuse their appreciations for the next day. The answer is yes, as long as you feel the appreciation deeply. However, for a loved one you know well, try to find new things to appreciate about the person, just to keep it fresh and interesting. For example, if you'd like your teenage son to remember to take the garbage out each week, you can express appreciation for his actions through Transformational Telepathy (or in person, of course), and it is very likely that he'll remember to do it more often.

Some people ask me how they should begin each sentence. Sometimes, to save time, I like to write at the top: "I appreciate you for . . . " and then list all the qualities underneath in an itemized list. But you don't have to stick to that format. You can make it more conversational. Here's a fictional example:

Helen, I appreciate you for how much you care about your pets. You treat your dogs like they are people, and I can see how happy they are. I love the way you sing to them and call them your "children."

I totally respect you for all the years of university you went through, all the hard work you put into making a difference in people's lives as a medical doctor. I appreciate you for all those nights you had to stay up to tend to people in the ER and how you did your best to always have a smile on your face no matter what.

I appreciate you for how amazing you are at being a single mom—how you want the best for your child, and how you offer her a variety of experiences, including gymnastics, drumming, painting, and singing.

I really like the words *I appreciate you*, because there's less judgment connected with the word *appreciate*. In other words, you don't have to like or love the person, but you easily appreciate a quality about the person.

Here are some instances in which you can use Transformational Telepathy in your life:

- Resolving conflict with a person, a group, or a company
- Helping a loved one who is in trouble or who needs support
- Calming or comforting an insecure child or teen
- Before asking your boss for a raise
- Increasing harmony and efficiency in your workplace
- Nurturing long-distance relationships

- Increasing love and emotional intimacy in a romantic relationship

I have found that Transformational Telepathy works 100 percent of the time when resolving a conflict quickly. I can't tell you how many times I have used this when I have been upset over a misunderstanding or disagreement with someone. I've gotten so good at doing this out loud that I rarely have to write the list anymore. For example, I might take a bath or get comfy in my bed and start thinking out loud my appreciation of the person, as if they were in front of me. Sometimes, it is so real, I tear up. By the end of the telepathy session, I'm feeling calm, loving, and appreciative. Positive results usually show up within twenty-four to forty-eight hours for me.

In one instance, someone who was upset with me apologized the next morning for her behavior. In another instance, someone who wrote me an angry email ended up making a shift on her end and gave me a big smile and hug the next time I saw her. I wish you could've been there to witness the miracles.

Understand that Transformational Telepathy is something you do in private. You don't tell the other person that you're doing it, nor do they need to know. Sometimes your ego may want to step in and take credit for a positive shift or outcome. Contain your need for recognition. The Universe knows you've "done good" and that's all that matters. There will be side benefits to your life when you do this work, some that will seem miraculously synchronistic, so keep your heart open. It may or may not take thirty days for results to show, but for harmonious relationships of all types, doing this exercise daily is the best prescription.

Advanced Transformational Telepathy is something I teach in the Light Warrior Training Camp, as well as in the TOLPAKAN Healing Level 2 Practitioner Training Program. It involves more imagination and ingenuity in helping others to see your point of view and resonate more with you without resistance or manipulation. Often, you *get your way* and it turns out to be a beneficial outcome for all parties involved. For example, I've helped a client win her house back from a vindictive ex-husband. I've helped another woman get all her contractors to call her back after weeks of frustration, and I've helped yet another woman receive disability benefits after waiting months without any progress.

If you'd like to learn Advanced Transformational Telepathy, sign up for the next Light Warrior Training Camp live event and let me know what you'd like to shift. Details are in the Next Steps chapter.

Chapter Summary

1. Basic Transformational Telepathy is an easy technique that works well to increase harmony in relationships.

2. Conflicts may resolve in as little as twenty-four hours when you do this technique.

3. Doing this technique sends positive energy to other persons, releasing their resistance.

4. Don't be surprised if the other person has a 180-degree turnaround in their behavior soon after you start your thirty-day appreciation.

5. Doing Transformational Telepathy is like sending someone a packet of positive appreciation energy.

6. Advanced Transformational Telepathy is a more sophisticated technique to support your relationships by increasing resonance between two people so that the outcome is a win-win.

Chapter 9

Intuitive Impressioning

FEELING INTO FUTURE REALITIES

Intuitive Impressioning is a super-fun skill to learn. There are two ways in which I use it.

MAKING CHOICES

Intuitive Impressioning can be used to help make life choices. Another method is the muscle testing we've already discussed in Chapter 5. You can use the skill of Divine Muscle Testing to check which choice among a variety is for your highest good. Ask which option is most aligned with your Divine Path. Which path has the most Light? I call it *Light Path or Divine Path Scoring*. Divine Path Scoring is part of the TOLPAKAN Healing Method Level 2 Practitioner Certification; It is beyond what I can cover in this book.

So instead, Intuitive Impressioning is a Superpower method of accessing your intuition to make positive choices for yourself. Intuitive Impressioning is a completely different way of using your Superpowers, without muscle testing, to evaluate which path might be for your highest and greatest good.

As an example, say you are a college student and you don't have money to visit all the colleges to which you applied to inform your decision. You could do a left-brain logical exercise—in which you make a chart; write down the pros and cons of each college, including meal plans, professors, students, fun activities, geographical location, and so on—and *logically* make a conclusion.

However, that takes a lot of time. Or, you could use your right-brain, intuitive side to help you make the decision. Think of all the money you would save by not visiting all those campuses! With Intuitive Impressioning, you can visit these places without physically going there. Interested to learn how? Read on.

TUNE IN TO OTHERS

The second way that you can use Intuitive Impressioning is to tune in to how someone else feels, especially someone you may be having a problem or conflict with, or maybe a friend whose birthday is coming up.

You can use Intuitive Impressioning to tune in, for example, to how your boss at work feels and how he would receive your request for a raise. You could tune in to figure out what kinds of questions he would ask you or what his attitude might be or which day of the week might be better to ask for a raise.

Wouldn't that be cool? Well, you can do this, and it's not that difficult.

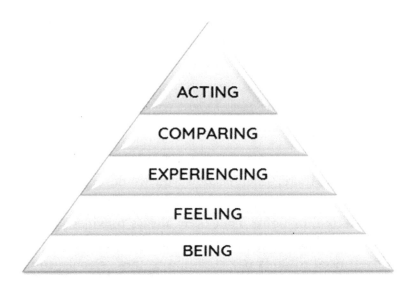

Intuitive Impressioning is done in five easy steps:

1. *Being* – in Stillness
2. *Feeling* – into the other person or situation
3. *Experiencing* – the future reality
4. *Comparing* – the different options
5. *Acting* – grateful and taking action based on your intuition

Step 1: *Being* in Stillness, which you've learned to do earlier in this book via STOIM, is the foundation from which you can access all your Superpowers, including your intuition. When you start in Stillness, your ego doesn't get in the way. Neither does your fear, nor your prejudices. By tuning in to your body through STOIM, it presses the Pause button on your ego-mind chatter, the chatter that encourages you to choose from a place of fear rather than a place of empowerment.

Step 2: Begin *feeling* into the person or situation you want more information about. In the example above, where you are trying to pick the right college to attend, you would feel into each of the colleges as if you were physically there, and tune in to how you feel, how the campus feels, how the people feel, even how the meal plan feels or tastes. Looking online at images of the campus can be helpful to evoke an emotion. In this case, I want you to feel *beyond* the image, pretending that you're really there.

Step 3: The next step is progressing from feeling to *experiencing*. You imagine yourself there. Imagine how you would enjoy being there. How do you feel emotionally? Calm? Joyful? Or do you feel shut down, contracted, or tight? Your body always provides you intuitive information, whether you perceive it or not and whether you like it or not. All you need to do is pay attention to these signals, so you can interpret them.

Generally speaking, sensations in the body that feel tight, cold, contracted, or unhappy are your body's way of saying no. Feelings of calm, joy, lightness, excitement, and expansion are your body's way of saying yes. Make friends with your body and pay attention to its signals. You can perceive an amazing amount of information this way. Remember, if you return too much to your critical mind, go back to STOIM and become grounded in Stillness once more.

If you have multiple choices ahead of you, take your time to tune in to each one individually, feeling and experiencing each of those choices, then interpreting your body's signals as to whether it's a yes or no.

Step 4: The next step is *comparing* the difference between how your body feels with one option versus another, depending on how many options you are entertaining. Tune in to your body to discern which option feels most calm, excited, blissed out, or enthusiastic. Any of those feelings and experiences are usually good signs you're on the right track. You may have to practice comparing because you may find several yesses, but only one is the best option. You're going to have to tune in to your own body to feel which one is the biggest yes.

On the other hand, you may have chosen a limited number of options that all feel *blah*. In other words, you're not really getting a big yes. In that case, you may need to do STOIM and ask yourself, in Stillness, if there are other choices you have not thought of. You may need to take a little break, drink some water, or walk outside in nature to become calm and grounded. At first, using Intuitive Impressioning to make big decisions can be difficult because so much is at stake. It may be best to start with smaller decisions first, such as: *Which restaurant should we go to for dinner tonight?* or *Which ice cream flavor do I really want?*

If you get a big shot of adrenaline, and your heart is pumping, and energy is flowing in your body, that can be excitement or fear. How do you tell the difference? I believe it depends on the scenes in your mind and how you interpret them. It also depends on whether you are tuning in to a place or a person. It is possible that the person you're feeling into may be in a place of fear, so temporarily, you feel their stuff. Don't worry about sponging this negative emotion, however, because with Intuitive Impressioning, your foundation is Stillness, where you are full of *you*.

Step 5: After you've done the comparing and you've made a decision, the last step in Intuitive Impressioning is *acting*. Acting on your intuitive information is a powerful way of telling the Universe that you mean business. If you don't act, it means you don't trust yourself or the Universe. Your intuition grows weaker with inaction. Your intuition grows stronger with positive action.

Every time you receive intuitive information and you act in alignment with that guidance, you reinforce the nervous system and those pathways, including the energetic pathways of being able to harness your intuition, to greater and greater degrees. With repetition, you'll be able to access it faster and faster, and it will be more dependable and reliable.

Here's a comparable scenario: A friend announces she is going to change her life. She tells her friends, family, and counselor that she knows she needs to get a divorce because she and her husband have irreconcilable differences. But week after week, month after month, nothing changes. She admits she needs the divorce but isn't taking any action to make it so. She keeps tolerating an intolerable situation at home. Sooner or later, everyone around her tunes her out. They don't believe her, and they've stopped listening to her.

It's like that with your intuition. If you don't take action, it's like your intuition will tune out and you won't be able to access it as easily. The good news is that the Universe will often confirm your positive choice with a sign or synchronicity, so be on the lookout for those.

Let's review Intuitive Impressioning for situations where you have multiple choices:

1. You bring yourself to a state of *being* in Stillness.

2. Then, you focus on *feeling* into each situation individually.

3. Practice *experiencing* each of them individually, imagining you're there; you're in that situation.

4. Once you've experienced each of them, begin *comparing* how your body feels and decide which one feels the best.

5. Now it comes time for *acting* on the one that feels the best to you, where you feel the calmest, or most joyful, or most expanded. That's usually the ideal choice.

How do you apply Intuitive Impressioning when working with other people? Intuitive Impressioning is super-handy when it comes to relationships. If you're reading this, you're probably a highly sensitive person and you might argue: *But Dr. Karen, I'm already feeling other people's stuff. I don't want to feel their stuff more!*

Well, I get it. Here's the thing: If you are indiscriminately feeling other people's stuff, that is indeed not a good thing. But you are learning to work with this gift so it is of benefit to you and those around you. Remember to cultivate good energetic boundaries. Regularly clear your energy field. Consistently practice BEING. These practices will help you *consciously* tune in to another person without problems. You will be able to pop in and pop out at will. You're not going sponge their emotions and "stuff." Got it?

I know I sound like a broken record, but please make sure that before you do Intuitive Impressioning on people, you've been practicing Stillness through STOIM, which keeps it safe and fun.

To walk you through how to do Intuitive Impressioning on people, let's take the example of wanting a raise at work. You want to know how to approach your boss at the right time, in the right way, so that they are more likely to say yes to you. The first step, of course, is *being* in Stillness.

Next, you're going to feel into your boss and that means picturing them in your mind and putting yourself in their proverbial shoes. Feel into their situation, their desires, their responsibilities. What makes them tick? What stresses them out? Who do they need to please? What's important to them? What do they worry about? What challenges have they been going through lately, either professionally or personally? And how does that feel for them?

And while you're *feeling*, you probably will get some hits about some of the challenges they're going through right now. Some of the questions they'll ask about why you want a raise may come up as well, so it will help you prepare for the conversation.

The one question you'll need to answer for your boss or anyone you want something from is, *What's in it for me?* Meaning, if your boss gives you a raise, what's in it for them? In your mind, you can begin explaining to your boss what benefits they or the company will receive when they give you that raise. You can even imagine your boss listening intently and feeling good about giving you that raise.

In my live event, you learn Level 2 Transformational Telepathy, in which you positively influence how the boss feels about you asking for a raise. Teaching this skill requires face-to-face instruction, but in the meantime, you can do Level 1 Transformational Telepathy and write down ten things you appreciate about your boss for thirty days straight before you ask for that raise.

Remember, feel into your boss to learn what concerns they have. You're going to answer what's in it for them. The next step is to imagine the *experience* of a perfectly peaceful interaction for both you and your boss. From this grounded place of Stillness, continue to imagine which days of the week might be best. Feel into how you can catch your boss at the optimal time for both of you.

Now, don't let this be an excuse of not asking for a raise, because there may not be a perfect time, but there may be a relatively better time. Listen to your intuition.

Once you've gathered all that information, you can skip the next step, which is *comparing*, because you're not really comparing two situations unless you wish to create two scenarios of how to address the raise with your boss and comparing which one feels lighter and calmer to you. Once you have that information, write it down, just to make sure that all your talking points are very clear.

Finally, as you end your Intuitive Impressioning session, go back into STOIM and feel full of yourself—by this I mean not in the sense of being arrogant, but by allowing yourself to feel fully *you*. That way, any residual energies related to feeling into another person are dissolved. At this point it is up to you to take the appropriate *action* based on your intuition.

Intuitive Impressioning is just like any other practice. The skills you choose to practice will improve. If you're a basketball player, and you're learning to put the ball in the basket, and you practice free throws every day for ten minutes, you're going to get a heck of a lot better at doing free throws than someone who hasn't practiced at all. Michael Jordan, arguably the best basketball player that ever lived, had to put in hours of practice before he made it onto the varsity team in high school. He was too short and couldn't dunk a ball. Although he was disappointed and cried over the decision, Jordan practiced his skill day after day, not knowing if he'd get any taller. The rest is history. If he hadn't practiced, he wouldn't be where he is today.

With practice, you will get better at Intuitive Impressioning. It can be fun and rewarding when you can feel into what your mother would appreciate as a holiday or birthday gift, or say the exact, right words to comfort a sad friend. I have heard the words, *That's so very thoughtful of you!* so many times in my life, I've lost count. The funny thing is, it isn't *thought* that helped me guess what someone needed, it was *feeling*.

You can use Intuitive Impressioning for a whole host of things, like choosing a holistic health practitioner or choosing what to have for dinner. How about choosing a vacation spot for you and your family? Or discovering whether your kids would enjoy racing down rapids in a raft? You get the picture.

If you have children, I encourage you to teach them Intuitive Impressioning because they will be able to quickly assimilate this ability and apply it to all areas of their life, including their school life and their relationships. One client said she taught her daughter how to tap her intuition to make decisions, and now her daughter no longer bugs her incessantly with questions she can answer herself. It's empowering and it's freeing.

Chapter Summary

1. Intuitive Impressioning is a skill that doesn't require muscle testing and helps you make choices aligned with your Divine Path for your highest and greatest good.

2. Intuitive Impressioning can be used to tune in to another person so that you can optimize your relationship and your interactions.

3. Be centered in Stillness when you start and when you end your Intuitive Impressioning session, the latter especially when you're feeling into a person, so that you do not unintentionally continue feeling someone else's stuff.

4. It's vital for you to act upon intuitive information that you're given, even though it might be a little scary at first, because taking action hones your intuition and signals the Universe that you mean business.

Chapter 10

Healing by Proxy-Prop

REMOTE HANDS-ON HEALING FOR BEGINNERS

Reiki and other forms of hands-on energy healing have become incredibly popular over the last few decades, with throngs of people attending workshops all over the world to learn them. Hands-on healing methods are indeed wonderful. I have both given and received multiple modalities of energy healing.

Here's the thing. Not everyone wants to train as a professional energy healer, own an office, set up a massage table, and purchase malpractice insurance just to do hands-on energy healing. At least in the United States, and in some other areas of the world, there have been crackdowns on people doing healing because regulators are fearful that they're practicing medicine.

Let's be very clear. We are not practicing medicine anywhere in this book and definitely not through Healing by Proxy-Prop. We are helping people to balance their energy field and supporting their natural healing process.

Another issue with hands-on energy healing, in a practical sense, is that unless you are a licensed practitioner, such as a medical doctor, naturopath, or chiropractor, problems can arise if you physically touch another person during a healing, depending on the laws in your region. During a healing session, the altered consciousness that results can put both practitioner and client at risk if, for instance, sexual energies arise.

Another problem is that people who have been sexually traumatized, abused, or harassed—and that's 25 percent of women and 7 percent of men in according to one study[19]—may feel unexpectedly uncomfortable in the middle of a session if these memories resurface when being physically touched by a healer, even in a nonsexual way. Honestly, it took me years to trust a male chiropractor or massage therapist enough to work on me because of inherited traumas that caused me to fear men, although I do not have a past history of sexual abuse. Many survivors of any kind of trauma carry with them Post Traumatic Stress Disorder, or PTSD, which affects the parasympathetic nervous system. They, too, may respond to triggers unexpectedly and uncomfortably.

Healing by Proxy-Prop is a way in which you can do profound energy healing on others without physically touching another person. You can even do healing on yourself this way.

How do we do it? We use a prop.

Let me define some terms for you first. The word *proxying*, in the healing sense, means that there's something or someone who has taken the place of the person who is the subject of your healing. Now, in Healing by Proxy-Prop, we're using a prop as the proxy as opposed to a living, breathing person.

For example, if a child was in a coma in the hospital and you didn't have access to her, you could, with permission, do healing through the mother as a proxy.

19 Kearl, H. "The facts behind the #metoo movement: A national study on sexual harassment and assault." Stop Street Harassment: Reston, VA, 2018. stopstreetharassment.org/wp-content/uploads/2018/01/Full-Report-2018-National-Study-on-Sexual-Harassment-and-Assault.pdf

In Healing by Proxy-Prop, we're not using a human being, we are using a stuffed animal or doll as a prop. Yes, don't laugh, it works in our live Light Warrior Training Camp, where we pair up to do these healings on each other. I find it fascinating to watch people who have never before done any sort of hands-on energy healing receive amazing positive feedback from their volunteer subjects. The newbie healers are shocked, awed, and in tears because they created a positive impact on the other person the very first time they performed energy healing.

You might now be asking, "How big a doll or stuffed animal do I need?" Well, it's really up to you. Sometimes I find it helpful to have something sizeable enough so that I can move my hands around it easily. But it doesn't really matter. A prop that is larger than the size of your two hands combined would be ideal, because a lot of people like using both hands. But you can use something the size of one hand as well.

When I was a child, I owned a Holly Hobbie rag doll, and she was fairly big, about sixteen inches in height. That's the perfect size to proxy for a person. The prop you use should look like a human, having a head, arms, and legs. Obviously, you don't need a tail, but it's not a big deal if you have a teddy bear with a tail. So as long as it looks somewhat humanoid, then it'll be easy to use as a prop.

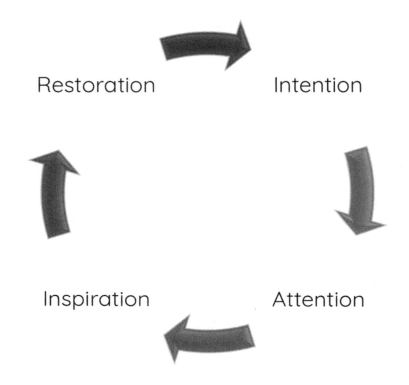

Let's cover the four steps of Healing by Proxy-Prop on another person:

1. *Intention* – set an intention to heal and harmonize.
2. *Attention* – pay attention to energy flowing in your hands.
3. *Inspiration* – let inspiration in the Stillness guide the movement of your hands.
4. *Restoration* – feel the sense of balance and harmony through your hands.

What about the other person, the subject, during the healing? Before beginning the session, it's good to suggest to the recipient that they be in a state of receiving. It doesn't mean that they're not receiving your healing even if they're at work. But I believe that they're going to feel much better if they can pay attention to their bodies while you're performing the healing.

Prepare the person you are helping:

1. Schedule a thirty-minute session with them during which they can be receptive.

2. Ask them to describe their symptoms and help you set a healing intention.

3. Instruct them that their job during this session is to relax while lying down or seated and observe how their body feels.

Step 1: After you've asked permission to perform a healing on the other person and clarified what result they desire, you set the *intention* that healing will occur in the highest and best way, with grace and ease, letting go of any attachment to outcome. If this person is under the age of eighteen, you will need to ask permission of their legal guardian and record that you have their permission. And if you are doing a Healing by Proxy-Prop on someone other than the person who asked you for the healing, you will need to get permission from the adult recipient to be fully ethical.

Step 2: After you've set an intention to heal and harmonize, rub your hands together to get the energy flowing, and focus your *attention* on what your hands are feeling after rubbing them together. You should be feeling movement or energy in your hands. That's just to get you used to feeling energy flow. In the future, you may notice that simply paying attention to your hands may start the flow of energy without needing to rub them together.

Step 3: Let your *inspiration* guide how to move your hands over the prop, keeping in mind the intention to heal and harmonize. If the recipient has told you they are experiencing knee pain, for example, you might move your hand in and around or over the knee area of this prop. However, let your inspiration guide where your hands want to move. Being in Stillness helps you refine your Superpower senses.

Even if the person reports having left knee pain, you might be inspired to move your hand down the spine. Feel and observe what happens to the energy in your hands as you pass by parts of the proxy. Maybe you feel a spot that doesn't have any energy. Maybe you'll want to use your hands to even out that low-energy area. Alternatively, maybe another area feels too hot or active to you, and you are inspired to disperse the excess energy.

You are harmonizing the person's energy fields with your hands. As if you are sculpting a piece of beautiful pottery, smooth out areas with holes or jaggedness until you feel there is nothing else to smooth out.

You can move your hands in whatever way feels right for you. Make sure that you are comfortable, whether you're sitting or standing. If you need to take a break and adjust your position, it's perfectly fine. Continue when you are ready.

Remember to breathe! Some people hold their breath when they are concentrating too hard. Let things flow and relax as you facilitate the healing.

You will get a sense, and it could be within three minutes or thirty minutes, that your work is finished when the energy feels smooth to you. When it feels harmonized, there's nothing else to do.

Step 4: At this point, you'll feel a sense of restoration, which is the last and final step. You're feeling in your hands that everything is balanced and restored to harmony. You can then end the session and thank the prop and the Universe for its role in the healing process. I often like to close my hand in the prayer position and bow my head.

In Reiki class, we used to draw a two half circles with each hand, meeting in the middle, before the closing our hands in prayer with the intention of closing the energy field and energetically separating from the prop and the recipient. You can make up your own closing ritual, whatever feels right for you. Or you can go back into Stillness, where you are back to being sovereign and feeling fully like yourself.

That's it. Very simple instructions.

You can perform Healing by Proxy-Prop in a separate location from the recipient.

After you're done, you can call them to debrief. Let's say you are helping your Aunt Janie in Florida and you're in Tennessee. Now, here's where the ego can be a problem early on in your healing practice.

You do the session, and she says she didn't feel anything. It doesn't mean that you didn't do it right or didn't help her situation. Don't take it personally. Some people aren't grounded in their bodies. They don't practice the BEING state. On the other hand, sometimes they'll feel a lot going on and that might make your ego swell. Whatever feedback you hear, remain neutral. Trust that the Universe did the healing in the best way possible, and be grateful.

If you're doing multiple healing sessions over a period of time, you might want to write down the feedback so you can track the changes and look for trends.

AFTER THE SESSION

Healing by Proxy-Prop is helpful for both parties. First, you get practice performing the healing as well as being nonattached to the result. Second, it's helpful for the other person because they get a chance to receive and get connected to their bodies through attention.

It's possible they might fall asleep because they're so relaxed, and that's okay. Let them know that if they, for whatever reason, have difficulty feeling any energy moving, it is completely okay, whatever was done was for the highest good. Invite them to give you feedback on how they feel in a few days. Instruct them to rest and drink plenty of water.

You may wish to share with them that it's possible they may experience a detoxification or healing reaction. This is a natural and self-limited stage during the process of healing wherein they may experience temporary discomfort, either physically or emotionally. Making the intention that the healing be done with grace and ease may prevent these symptoms.

Please note that knowing Healing by Proxy-Prop *does not give you permission to be a professional healer.* This is not a certification of any type, and it would be unethical to receive money in exchange for these healings unless you are already certified in some other modality that allows it. There are a lot of rules and ethics involved in becoming a professional healer, and this is beyond what I can teach in this book. But the cool thing is that this technique is a fantastic, empowering way to help close friends and family.

You might want to know: *Who is actually doing the healing, if not me?* Personally, I believe we are the conduits of healing, meaning that we aren't doing the healing per se. You could also see us as directors of energy, with the Universe, or our Spirit/God teams doing the actual work. Who knows for sure? As long as you have good intentions, and come from a place of unconditional love and Stillness, you will only help others, never harm them.

So how do you do Healing by Proxy-Prop for yourself?

It's pretty easy. Make an intention that the proxy—in this case, the teddy bear or doll—is you. It's a degree of separation that really helps some people do self-healing in an effective way. Sometimes when we focus on ourselves too intently, we can get too attached, but if we are focusing our attention on the proxy, we can more easily let go and experience the energy.

Remember to go through the same steps: Set an intention to heal and harmonize all parts of yourself. Rub your hands and put your attention on the energy flowing through your hands. Then move your hands over the prop, both feeling the energy and smoothing out the energy. Finally, sense when the restoration is complete, the energies are all smoothed out, and end the session as if you would for another person.

There you have it! You've learned hands-on healing.

Chapter Summary

1. Healing by Proxy-Prop is a great hands-on healing technique that does not require extensive training or malpractice insurance.

2. This method is safe and nonthreatening, especially to those who may find hands-on healing too intimate for them.

3. Before you do Healing by Proxy-Prop, remember to get permission.

4. You can self-heal by intending that the proxy is you instead of another person.

5. It's always advisable to go into Stillness, your BEING state, before and after your session.

6. Some hands-on healers use the technique of closing the circle with their hands, then close their hands in prayer and bow their heads in thanks, to separate energetically from the recipient and end the session.

Chapter 11

Perception Kung Fu

THE REFRAME RELIEVER™
AND OVERCOMING OBSTACLES

I have only recently realized something that is vitally important to our ability to manifest a life of joy, happiness, peace, and abundance: Our ability to be in the present moment and respond, rather than react, to life circumstances. When life throws us a curveball, I call it an *abundance challenge*. If you view these curveballs or challenges as the Universe providing you with an opportunity to grow, to achieve the same vibration as what you desire—whether that is more money, more clients, better health, or better relationships—it won't feel as uncomfortable.

You might be wondering why I'm calling the focus of this chapter *Perception Kung Fu*. I am a student of Wing Chun kung fu. Unlike most other popular kung fu styles, Wing Chun has been relatively unknown, until it was popularized in the film, *Ip Man*, a biographical account of the man who brought it to the West. Let me share a little bit about this martial art so you can see why I'm applying it to your Superpower training.

Wing Chun was developed, as the legend goes, by a Chinese female abbess or headmistress. She developed it out of necessity. She had to find a way to overcome the expert martial art tactics of fellow Shao Lin monks who had been recruited by warlords. She taught it to commoners who didn't have the luxury of decades of martial art study.

Many people are familiar with Shao Lin and various types of Shao Lin kung fu, but few people know about Wing Chun. I'm sharing this with you because it's significant that, in Wing Chun kung fu, there are no fancy high kicks or showy moves. In contrast, Wing Chun is all about grounding, relaxation, and the ability to manage angle and distance to beat your opponent. That's why a five-foot, one-hundred-pound woman can still win a fight with a six-foot, two-hundred-pound, muscular man.

Ip Man was one of the modern-day students of Wing Chun who became a master and brought it to the West. Bruce Lee was one of his pupils. Ip Man, like many Chinese men, was quite small in stature, yet had been known to win fights with men who were much taller and heavier than he was.

Perception Kung Fu is the ability to overcome a seemingly unsurmountable obstacle in your life with skills similar to those used in Wing Chun. When you desire what you do not already have, the Universe works to present you with opportunities to raise your vibration to match that which you desire. In doing so, the opposite or contrasting energy must show up for you to clear, heal, or overcome. A great analogy would be the story of *The Wizard of Oz*. In the story, Dorothy desires to return home to Kansas and ends up recruiting the lion, the tin man, and the scarecrow. Each one of them, including Dorothy, has a desired outcome, and each one of them encounters a challenge or obstacle. By learning to overcome the obstacle, each obtains their desire in the best way possible.

The story would have turned out quite differently if Glinda the Good had waved her magic wand, given each of them a handout, and solved their problems for them. None of the characters would have evolved. The lion would not have learned that he was already courageous, the tin man would not have appreciated that he was already loving and compassionate, and the scarecrow would not have understood that he was already resourceful and intelligent. And of course, Dorothy had to learn that she had everything she already needed to return home if she chose to.

You are each of these characters in the movie of your life. All these qualities of courage, heart, resourcefulness, and your ability to connect to Source (get home) are what you need to overcome any obstacle. Perception Kung Fu is the choice to change your perception from obstacle or unexpected event to a stepping stone to getting you to where you want to go.

Imagine that your goal is represented by an imaginary a pot of gold at the end of the street. You're walking toward it when, all of a sudden, a two-ton boulder drops right in the middle of your path. The boulder represents obstacles we experience in our lives. What do we as humans often do when something bad happens to us? Have you ever complained, "It's always two steps forward and one step back"? We resist it. We complain about it. We tell ourselves it shouldn't be there. Things shouldn't get in our way. We convince ourselves that the path should be smooth and not bumpy. Our beliefs, unfortunately, are myths stripping us of our inner joy and peace.

Resisting is like pushing against a two-ton boulder to move it off your path.

What could you do instead of pushing against it? You could choose to retreat, right? But what would happen if, every time an obstacle presented itself to you, you retreated? Would you be any closer to your pot of gold? Probably not.

What other options do you have? What if you learned how to climb that boulder? Would you be closer to your goal? What if you learned how to navigate around that boulder? Would that bring you closer to your goal? The answers are yes and yes.

You could spend all your energy getting pissed off at that boulder and telling everyone how awfully inconsiderate it was to show up on your path, or you could figure out a way to circumnavigate it in the most efficient way possible.

In Wing Chun kung fu, we manage an attacker coming at us as our obstacle to overcome. In the Light Warrior Training Camp, we give you an embodied experience of how you do Perception Kung Fu. *Spoiler alert!* I'll share how we train.

At the live event, I am the protagonist and one of the participants represents the goal at the other end of the room. As I am making my way toward my goal, my husband, James, poses as the antagonist in this scenario. He jumps in front of me, blocking my path. Now to make things more interesting, he's not just standing there. Instead, he lunges at me with a side kick!

I first demonstrate option one, which is blocking the kick the best I can while I'm staying in one spot. There are some benefits to being able to block a strike. First, if you practice blocking a lot of strikes, your body is going to be a lot stronger and more resilient. Your bones will probably end up denser, too, over time. Some martial artists train this way to get stronger.

However, for option one, there aren't just pros; there are cons. The cons to blocking a strike, or an obstacle in this case, is that it can be pretty painful. Unless you're in love with pain, it's not fun blocking, aka resisting, every obstacle that comes your way. Although you might become stronger in the long run, you'll first be banged up and bruised up. And guess what? *Resisting the obstacle never really moved you any closer to your goal.* Yet it probably made you more tired.

People often choose option one. They resist whatever is going on and they brace for impact. But what are some other options if resisting isn't getting you closer to your goals?

Your other option is to run away. You could back up. You could avoid the obstacle. You could *retreat*. Go in the opposite direction of the obstacle that is coming right for you. During my live event, I demonstrate this by jumping back when my husband, James, tries to kick me.

There are pros and cons to retreating, just as there are pros and cons to resisting. The benefit of retreating is that you're much less likely to get hurt, bruised, or banged up—that is, unless you miscalculate your distance. You might even become an expert at running away. The bad part about retreating is that you'll end up farther from your goal.

A lot of people react this way when they start toward a goal. An obstacle shows up, which it must, for you to get what you want. Many people think erroneously that abundance means you don't have to act. But let me tell you this: The Universe will grow you to the place that's a resonant match with what you want to achieve and what you want to accomplish. Obstacles train us to *choose* the right action that moves us closer to our goal. Retreating isn't a viable option when you're presented with an obstacle in your life. You can't avoid life.

If resisting is tiring and retreating is counterproductive, what other option do you have?

In Wing Chun kung fu, we avoid retreating. We might step back temporarily, but the technique we employ is to get close to our target by changing the angle of our bodies so that our center line is facing theirs, but their center line is no longer facing ours, and then stepping toward our opponent to attack.

During the live event, when James runs and kicks at me, instead of retreating or blocking the kick, I step toward him at an angle. Suddenly, I'm at an advantage and he is at a disadvantage. The kick has not only missed me completely, but I am in a position to attack him and I am much closer to my goal. As a side note, in this scenario, no blocking is necessary, but in Wing Chun, there are times when we block a hit and strike simultaneously.

Once I demonstrate all the different options of dealing with an obstacle, then participants try them. There is something magical about teaching this simple yet effective concept. Don't worry; they don't actually get hurt or kicked in these training exercises. Everyone in the class can clearly see that, with this technique, we do not get hit; we are in striking distance of the obstacle, and we are closer to the object of our desires or that pot of gold, so to speak.

When obstacles or things you don't like come your way, you have a choice. You can resist, or you can retreat, like most people do. Or you could *change your perception about the obstacle and respond—rather than react—to it.*

Let me say that a different way. To respond, not react, to life's circumstances, you need to change your perception. For everything that's happened in your life, especially when things aren't going as planned (or *as preferred*, as I like to say), respond rather than react and shift your perception. Then, you'll be closer to your goals. You'll also be in resonance with the frequency of abundance. This is analogous to shifting your angle in Wing Chun kung fu.

One of the greatest tools that you can use to execute Perception Kung Fu is something called the *Reframe Reliever.*

T. Harv Eker, bestselling author of *Secrets of the Millionaire Mind*, used to say in his live trainings that if you believe that whatever happens is there to serve you, then there is nothing that can get in your way. In other words, if you hold the belief: *Everything happens for a reason, and that reason is there to serve me*, you can choose it whenever "bad" things happen. This positive belief has been incredibly useful in my life.

The Reframe Relie

response rather thar

Receive

serve you. One of my favorite quote

Choices and Illusions: "I can't wai

Meaning that no matter wh

you.

To reframe the si

happening *to* v

great opport

new. Y

who

THI

There are three steps

or obstacle:

1. *Receive* the wisdom in Stillness.

2. *Reframe* with creativity and humor.

3. *Respond* from the highest perception possible.

Step 1: *Receive* the wisdom in the Stillness. Here, we're going back to Stillness because it is so foundational to your success. All answers are there and all the wisdom is there—your inner wisdom and your connection to Source. Your inner wisdom will drop in as you pay attention to the movement inside your body and as your mind stills. Whether you believe the inspiration or insight is from your angels, guides, Higher Self, or Source, it doesn't really matter. Be open to the possibility that the obstacle or setback may be of service to you or your goals. That alone will be enough to release resistance and let the flow of wisdom arise.

Step 2: *Reframe* the situation, using creativity and humor. This may include inventing stories about how this situation or obstacle might

...s is from Dr. Eldon Taylor's book,
...t to see what good comes out of this."
...at bad things happen, they can still serve

...uation, shift your perception from the situation
...ou to the situation happening to *serve* you. Here is a
...unity for you to learn, to evolve, or to experience something
...u may witness and appreciate how much you've evolved from
...you have been.

Step 3: You *respond* to the obstacle or situation based on your reframed perception. You respond with the highest vibration. Instead of reacting—mired in negative energy—you are responding from the highest place possible.

When you respond rather than react to circumstances in your life, you are at that moment creating your future reality. That future reality will either be harmonious or disharmonious based on whether you're responding or reacting.

Let me give you an example.

One of my good friends, Jake, woke up one day to discover his car was stolen. Not long before, Jake had studied my Unlock Your Superpowers Program, in which I discuss the concept of abundance challenges. At the moment he realized the car was stolen, he had a choice: he could either feel sorry for himself or he could reframe the experience. He chose to reframe it.

He realized that, in the past, he would have been depressed for weeks if something like this happened to him. But in this case, he chose not to go there. He was able to reframe the situation so quickly that he did a Facebook livestream celebrating how undisturbed he was that his car was stolen. He shared how he surprisingly wasn't sad, depressed, or angry about the situation. He was looking on the bright side.

"I'm healthy," he said; "I'm alive. Yeah, my car got stolen. But I know someone's going to lend me their bike to get to work."

And sure enough, somebody did.

Jake was able to let go of expectations and was open to whatever was supposed to happen for his highest good. In this case, it was the Universe showing him how much he had changed in a short period of time, and he was joyful about his evolution.

Jake had passed his abundance challenge with flying colors, and I had a pretty strong feeling that he was going to get his car back intact, even though he was not attached to the outcome. A couple weeks went by, and he got a call from the police. They found his car under, apparently, very unusual circumstances.

The couple who had stolen the car had been experiencing some mechanical trouble, so they stopped at a gas station to try to figure out what was wrong. The two of them ended up getting into a fight. The woman was hitting the passenger-side window with a solid object, but the window would not shatter. Alarmed, the gas station attendant called the police. When the police came, they ran the plates and discovered it was a stolen vehicle. The couple was arrested, and Jake got his car back.

If that wasn't miraculous enough, get this: When Jake got the car back, he found out that the car's brake lines had ruptured, which is why the thieves had stopped at the gas station. It was easily fixed for $50. Jake felt relief to know that he wasn't driving the car when the brake lines ruptured. Who knows what would have happened?

That's a perfect example of how he was able to reframe a bad situation. Not only did he have the opportunity to witness how far he had come emotionally and spiritually, he got his car back without a scratch. Neat, eh?

Want some fun practice with the Reframe Reliever?

Do the Reframe Reliever for each of the following scenarios. Make up the reason why it may be for your highest and greatest good.

- You just got fired from your job.

- Your husband just left you.

- You sprain your ankle.

- Your teenage daughter just told you she is pregnant.

- You just got diagnosed with cancer.

- Your house burnt down when you and your family were on vacation.

Some of these may be challenging, especially if it hits close to home. If you need community support around any of them, please reach out to our social media Light Warrior Network (link in Next Steps).

Chapter Summary

1. Perception Kung Fu is a way to view anything uncomfortable coming into your life as something that serves you.

2. Using Stillness, you can extract your inner wisdom and reframe the situation to perceive it as being for your highest and greatest good.

3. Responding rather than reacting to a situation increases your vibration and your ability to create a future reality more in alignment with your desires.

4. Practice the Reframe Reliever whenever you can, and feel free to reach out to my private online community if you need some support.

SECTION 3
CREATING

Chapter 12

STOIM for Masterful Manifesting

HOW TO CREATE YOUR IDEAL FUTURE REALITY

Now that you have a sense of how to truly *be* through STOIM, we can use this awareness, attention, and skill to help you create an amazing new reality—one that you would love to experience. Most people run around each day completely unconscious of what they are thinking or feeling; however, our nervous systems are constantly broadcasting what we desire to the Universe. The Universe delivers it to us through a *resonance match*. A resonance match means that the Universe will help you manifest a future reality based on your core resonance or vibration.

When you are in Stillness, that resonance is the true *you*, your core being. When you resonate at your true core being, beautiful and wonderful circumstances arise—abundance of all types: abundant health, abundant wealth, abundant love, and so on. These events and qualities become gravitationally attracted to you. You create new realities based on that resonance. In the quantum world, we might describe it as *jumping to another quantum stream of reality*.

In this chapter, STOIM for Masterful Manifesting, you learn to use that access to Zero Point in Stillness for manifesting your greatest dreams. I hope you are as excited as I am!

One of my wealth teachers, T. Harv Eker, used to say in his workshops that the reason people don't get what they want is because they don't know what they want. For the most part, he is right. When I work with clients from all over the world and from all walks of life, I ask them to describe their ideal future reality. Guess what? Many of them are not able to express what it looks like or feels like. Many of them are trapped into thinking their current reality is the only reality that exists. It takes a bit of coaching to guide them to connect with their ideal future reality.

Imagine that you have a GPS device in your car. You turn on the GPS and start driving. Does the GPS give you any information or directions if you don't plug in your destination?

No. The GPS will track you and display where you are relative to space and Earth, but without a destination, it can't give you any directions. Manifesting your wants or desires is similar. You must have a clear vision of your desired outcome to manifest it. If you focus 99 percent of your conscious waking time on your current reality, that's the past. The next moment passes, and the next, and the next. You're re-manifesting the past.

You can't affect your future if you haven't created it in your mind first. That's how it works in the quantum reality. Gregg Braden, in his books and in the TV series *Missing Links*, shared a story about a Hopi Indian friend of his whose village had been suffering a severe drought. He invited Gregg to accompany him to a sacred site to pray for rain. Gregg was incredibly excited because he thought he was going to learn some special Hopi Indian technique to make it rain.

He hiked with his friend, David, up to a sacred site. There was a stone circle on the ground. His friend motioned to him to wait as he did his prayer. His friend stood inside the stone circle, closed his eyes, honored his ancestors, and in less than a minute, he walked back to Gregg and said, "I'm hungry. Let's go get a bite to eat."

At this point, Gregg was quite perplexed because he didn't really understand what just happened. He asked his friend, "I thought you were going to pray for rain?"

His friend revealed this is the traditional way the Hopi manifest rain. David described it with great detail to Gregg. He said that when he closed his eyes, he experienced what it would look like, feel like, and smell like when his village was deluged with rain. Then to end the prayer, David gave thanks of gratitude and appreciation. Gregg concluded that the *feeling* is the prayer, not the words we say or even the thoughts in our mind.

In the Weather Magic chapter, you'll see what we teach is similar to the Hopi way.

When I was a child, I used prayers of supplication, pleading with God for help. Instead, this is more like feeling grateful and thanking God that the outcome has already manifested.

Do you remember hearing this growing up? "Ask and ye shall receive." Gregg shared that the original text (as reported by author Neil Douglas-Klotz in *Prayers of the Cosmos: Meditations on the Aramaic Words of Jesus*) says:

All things that you ask straightly, directly . . . from inside my name, you will be given. So far you have not done this. Ask without hidden motive and be surrounded by your answer. Be enveloped by what you desire, that your gladness be full.

By being "enveloped by what you desire," you resonate at the frequency of your desires when you experience your new reality and give thanks for it through your feelings, which are your sensitivity Superpowers.

Now, it's your turn to create your future new reality. First, be clear on what you want. Don't worry. You're allowed to change your mind. Every time you make a new choice, however, the wheels of the Universe start moving you in a new direction. Remember, setting your goals—your ideal new reality—is like setting a GPS. For example, you can set your GPS for London, England, but if you change your mind halfway there, and set your GPS to New Zealand, you'll be taking a new course. Small adjustments mean small detours. Large adjustments mean large detours. Make sense?

Here are tips on how to write down your new future reality in a way that makes manifesting more effective:

Tip #1: Write your new reality as if it's happening now or has already happened. In other words, use present or past tense in your language. Avoiding writing in future tense because that means it's happening in the future. If you write it using present tense, you can get into the feeling that it is happening now. If you write it using past tense, you can celebrate the feeling of having already accomplished it.

Tip #2: Use descriptive words that inspire you and rev you with good energy. For example, instead of writing something like: *I am healthy* or, *My body is healthy*, you might want to write something like: *My body is radiantly healthy, and I am consistently landing double axel jumps.* You want to use high-vibrational, positive words such as *vibrant, radiant, joy*. A fun exercise can be simply writing down words that really inspire you.

Tip #3: Be specific about what you desire. If you express an outcome that is Plain-Jane, it's like directing your car's GPS to "Go to the mountains" without naming which ones. Your GPS probably won't progress very far with those instructions. When you are vague, the Universe has a creative way of giving you feedback. Sometimes you discover more precisely what you don't want.

On the other hand, some people might be so specific they block the Universe from creating the best outcome. I'll give you an example. When I was working in a molecular biology lab in medical school at the University of Ottawa, there was a security guard who would come by and say hello. I'll call him Jerry. Now, Jerry was a large fellow who definitely looked like he had eaten one too many doughnuts, but he was super-friendly and talkative, so I got to chat with him on many occasions.

He kept saying he was going to marry a "Kim Basinger," meaning a woman who looks like the actress from the movie *9½ Weeks*, which was popular at the time. I questioned him about this. And at the time, I didn't really believe somebody who was an overweight security guard would be able to attract a hottie like Kim Basinger.

I said to him, "How important is it that she look like Kim Basinger?"

And he said, "Well, very important." He gave me strict criteria: she had to be blonde and have bust-waist-hip measurements of 35-24-35.

That didn't sit well with me at the time, being a feminist and all. He only focused on her looks. Maybe the perfect person for him might be a redhead or maybe someone who's a little taller or someone who's got a bigger bust size, for example. *How could he limit himself to such a shallow description?* I thought to myself.

I know more now than I did then. There was nothing wrong with Jerry's criteria, per se, if that's what he truly desired. But most of us desire happiness. By limiting the Universe to giving him one specific vision of outer appearances, Jerry limited his chances of manifesting true love. If marrying a Kim Bassinger look-alike was aligned with Jerry's Divine Path and would create true happiness, then the Universe *would* conspire to co-create that reality with him.

When considering your ideal future reality, write down specifics about what's important to you, but leave other details open so the Universe can pleasantly surprise you.

I asked the Universe to manifest my perfect, ideal, dream love-partner, and I thought I was being specific enough. I told the Universe I wanted a skater. I wanted someone who was as good a skater as I was because I absolutely loved pair skating, and I really missed my former pair skating partner who had moved away.

At the time, I was having a lot of fun with Doreen Virtue angel cards, so I would do intuitive readings for myself. Because I was so determined to manifest my ideal partner, I had taken Laura Day's workshop called "The Circle" and read her book about how to manifest. I had spent almost a year trying hard to manifest this man into my life. However, I had neglected to clear the space for my ideal partner. Interestingly, every time that I pulled the angel cards out, I'd choose a card that said, "You're not asking for what you truly want." After picking this card on multiple occasions, I got pretty fed up. One time, I decided to be obnoxiously cheeky, and wrote down *everything*. Yup, I wrote down everything I wanted in my ideal partner, including his ideal pair skating height, his good looks, and his penchant for chopping wood and mowing the lawn!

You can read the gory details in my eBook, *Creating Your Fairy Tale Love Life: How to Harness the Law of Attraction to Attract Your Dream Partner*. Up until that point, because I didn't believe I could manifest a figure skating partner who was also a love partner, I didn't actually write it down. That was the clincher. I was too scared to ask for what I wanted, so I was settling for something less. The Universe was teaching me to *go for it*.

I finally let loose and asked for exactly what I wanted. As soon as I created the space for the Universe to manifest my ideal partner, I met James. He was everything I asked for and more. The Universe didn't bring me a figure skater, because there were none who matched my criteria. Instead, it brought me an inline skater who was talented enough to learn figure skating in half the time I did. We have since won multiple national and international medals in adult skating, and I'm having the time of my life.

You might want to set up a special creation date when you enjoy writing your ideal future reality by yourself or with a trusted friend or partner. Put on some fun music, make sure you feel good while you're writing it, maybe have some candles going, some twinkly lights, whatever makes you feel good and special about this new reality you're creating from scratch from your imagination.

Once you have the template of your new reality and can clearly envision it, remember the Universe will deliver it in the coolest, best way possible. It's usually not even imaginable by our human standards. When you've accomplished this, you are ready for STOIM for Masterful Manifesting.

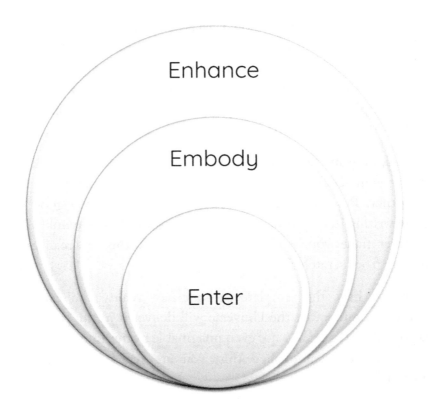

To use STOIM for Masterful Manifesting, there are three steps:

1. *Enter* Stillness.

2. *Embody* your ideal new reality

3. *Enhance* and elevate your emotions.

Step 1: *Enter* your state of being, your STOIM, and enjoy that space. Focus, feel, and follow the flow, as per usual.

Step 2: *Embody* that new, ideal reality by seeing, feeling, and observing all the senses of your physical body, as if it's happening to you now or has already happened.

Step 3: Last, *enhance* and elevate your emotions and feelings to a higher vibrational state.

After you enter STOIM and you're resonating at that peaceful place, you're then going to tune in or insert your ideal new reality. You're going to imagine it and embody it with all fibers of your being. It's happening right now. If you're wondering whether you have the capability to do this, the answer is a resounding yes! We all have that capability. We often use our imaginations for less than optimal things. For example, we get anxious about bad things that might happen. We get so worked up about it, our nervous systems respond as if they are happening now, even though they're imagined.

We are also affected by past trauma, grief, and so on. The minute we tune in to past trauma, our emotions and body can start resonating at that lower vibration. In STOIM for Masterful Manifesting, you harness your creative powers and redirect the flow to create your new ideal reality rather than rehash old anxiety-producing realities.

There's a quote attributed to Malachy McCourt that I really resonate with. "If you have one foot in the past and one foot in the future, you're pissing on the present." By embodying your new reality in the *now*, you are creating your new ideal reality in the future.

To embody your new reality, you don't have to experience everything contained in that reality. Picture a scene in which you're feeling great and enjoying life. See it in your mind and then feel it in your body. Where are you? What's the temperature there—cold, hot? Is it rainy? Is it sunny? Is there wind?

Feel with your mind's eye, and then listen, and hear. What do you hear? What are the sounds in your new reality? Are children giggling? Waves lapping the shore?

Imagine what you smell. Maybe you're in downtown Florence, Italy, and smelling beautiful scents wafting from restaurants. And then taste. Imagine what you're eating (if you happen to love food like I do).

Step 3, in which you enhance and elevate your emotions, is like jet fuel for your rocket of manifestation. It propels your manifestation. Another way to enhance and elevate our emotions is to celebrate. I also call it doing a "happy dance of thanks."

In one of the trainings that I did at the Olympic Training Center in Lake Placid, New York, with some of the winter athletes, I had them practice celebrating winning the Olympics. I suggested the scenario to focus on. They were to close their eyes and visualize their best performance, taking first place and winning the Olympic gold medal. And when they opened their eyes, we all stood up, and I instructed them to celebrate by hooting and hollering as loud as they could, as if they were really there. It was amazing. The emotions skyrocketed and the room filled with electrifying joy. Almost everybody felt it. I say *almost everybody* because there was one person who was an outlier. She had a really hard time with the exercise.

She wasn't really willing to give the exercise her all. My sense was that she was too embarrassed to celebrate "ahead of time." And unfortunately, although she did make it to the Olympics, she performed poorly in her sport and was not in medal contention. On the other hand, one of the bobsledders, who was able to celebrate easily, suffered a broken bone (Abundance Challenge) and missed the Olympics, but fought back to win a gold medal at the World Cup months later. Who had the more desired result? I would argue it was the bobsledder. I wonder whether the other athlete would have placed higher if she had been willing to *practice* winning.

In Step 3, stretch yourself and enhance your emotions and senses by whatever means possible, such as dancing to rock-and-roll music in your living room, taking a hot bath with flowers and scented candles, or going out in nature and dunking in a lake. Do whatever makes you feel really good. That's the key.

By seeding Stillness with your desired quantum reality, including embodiment and emotion, you are choosing a desired "quantum stream" out of the myriad of potential quantum realities. The more often you seed Stillness, aka Zero Point, with your ideal new reality, the more your dominant resonance will change to reflect that which you desire.

Eventually, you'll be able to tune in to your new reality in an instant, without having to close your eyes or dance around your living room. Your nervous system will be so practiced in Stillness, you will able to resonate your new reality in a millisecond. Isn't that exciting?

Happy manifesting!

I like to say: *What we celebrate, we accelerate!* so every week in my private group on social media, we do *Win Wednesdays*, where you can practice celebrating your weekly wins and we can celebrate with you.

Chapter Summary

1. You can feed the Stillness or Zero Point with your ideal reality. In doing so, you choose a quantum stream that is aligned with your greatest dreams.

2. It's important to know what you want and record it clearly using passionate words to describe your reality as it is happening now or has happened in the past.

3. Remember to be specific but not overly controlling in your intention so the Universe can give you the best option as quickly as possible in the best way possible.

4. Remember the three steps to masterful manifesting: 1) entering Stillness, 2) embodying your new reality, and 3) enhancing your emotions.

5. Do STOIM for masterful manifesting every day, and become comfortable feeling those positive emotions while in your new reality.

6. Practice STOIM throughout your day, even if only for a few moments at a time, to anchor your positive new reality.

Chapter 13

Weather Magic

HOW TO INFLUENCE THE WEATHER

In this chapter, you learn to create the weather you want. Is that cool or what? Don't freak out because you're worried you might make a mistake. The Universe will not let you do anything that is harmful to another person, even if you're having a bad day.

Weather Magic will only work if it is for the highest and greatest good. Sometimes Mother Earth needs to rebalance herself, and if that means a major storm, no amount of Weather Magic will change that. Here's an example to illustrate more of what I mean. Say you desire fourteen days of sunny dry weather, but the farmers in your area desperately need rain. Your Weather Magic may produce mixed results in that you'll get sun during the day and rain only at night so you and the farmers can both be happy.

Weather Magic is really fun because you can change the quality of your life and other peoples' lives by using the abilities you already have within you. You can learn to harness those abilities and hone them for this particular goal.

I discovered Weather Magic in 2016 when I got an email from Kaitlyn Keyt, CEO of the VibesUp Company. I'm on her email list and I enjoy many of her products. On an odd Friday night, I was guided to read an email from her—I normally do not open my emails on date night, however, for whatever reason, I was checking my email.

Around 8:00 p.m., I saw Kaitlyn's email to all her subscribers asking us to pray for the people of Mexico. I had no idea what was going on because I don't watch the news—I usually tell my patients not to watch the news either—because it's full of drama and negative energy. In this instance, she was talking about a 216 mile-per-hour hurricane called Patricia that was hitting the shores of Mexico and was about to devastate an impoverished area. Thousands of lives were at stake.

I thought to myself: *That's interesting. I wonder why I opened this email?*

I had done successful Weather Magic before, but this time, I decided to ask my students to do it with me. I created a Facebook post and asked my Holistic Health Transformation students—of whom there were only about twenty at the time—to do some weather magic with me. I didn't give them the kind of detailed instruction that I'm going to give you in this chapter, but I basically told them to change the storm and save the people of Mexico using their imagination. What I saw in my mind as I did the Weather Magic was the hurricane petering out to a rain storm. And that's pretty much how I pictured it. Pretty simple, right?

We performed Weather Magic each on our own that Friday evening. By the next morning, I had forgotten about it. I went about my day as if nothing happened and was excitedly preparing for my friend's annual Halloween bash.

That night, after my husband and I had come back from the Halloween party, he said to me, "It worked!"

"What worked?" I asked.

"Your Weather Magic! It worked!"

"Oh, my gosh, I totally forgot about the hurricane, what's going on?"

"From the look of the news reports, that storm petered out, and now it's only rain."

The reports confirmed that weather magic is awesome and is for real.

Since then, I have asked many of my students, clients, and patients to do weather magic. And it's been really fun. For example, people have cleared clouds and rain for their son or daughter's wedding. I did that for a friend of mine who had her wedding on a mountaintop. Other people have cleared weather that was interfering with their trip or vacation. We have moved or changed the direction of storms, including multiple hurricanes. We have made it rain in areas of Australia that were devastated by fire.

Let me share with you how this works and how to harness the power within you to change the weather.

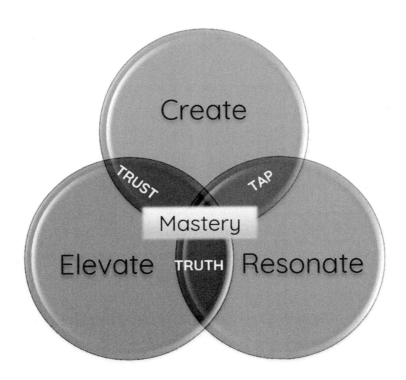

There's a three-step process to create the weather you want. You'll note that these steps are very similar to the Enter, Embody, Enhance steps in STOIM for Masterful Manifesting from the last chapter, just described slightly differently. The labels aren't as important as the concepts, so use whichever is easier for you to remember.

1. *Create* – the image of weather
2. *Resonate* – the feeling
3. *Elevate* – your emotions

Step 1. *Create* the ideal weather in your mind. See it in your mind and experience it in your mind.

Step 2: *Resonate* that new reality with all your senses and embody it as if it's happening right now in this moment.

Step 3: *Elevate* your emotions. That means be grateful, happy, and joyful that you're experiencing the weather that you desire.

When you create and resonate on a high level, you *tap* your intuitive abilities. Humans are amazing because of our imagination. Sometimes we can imagine bad things happening to ourselves, and we make our emotions all riled up about it. Why not turn that talent on its head? Why not use our imagination for positive manifestation?

When you can resonate your new reality and elevate your emotions, you learn the *truth* of who you really are: a powerful being. When you can elevate and create, then you learn to *trust* that you have the power to change your life and the Universe has your back. All masters of positive manifestation use this formula to one degree or another. When used well and used consistently, you gain *mastery* over your life! Weather Magic is one of many perks of being a masterful manifester. And here's the good news: you alone can move a hurricane. But it's more fun with friends.

Weather Magic is a subject I have taught online for free. You may ask, "Why do you teach something so powerful for free?" I want people to understand without a doubt how powerful they really are. If you can successfully do Weather Magic and you can teach your five-year-old how to do it, think about how empowered they may feel. What if each person on Earth was able to fully step into their power? Do you believe more humans on this planet would thrive?

That's why I love to teach Weather Magic as a first step, because it's easy and because anyone can do it, even a child. If people knew they had the power to change the weather for the highest good, then they might begin to believe that they have the power to change their own lives and heal themselves from whatever ails them.

Let's view an example of how you could use your imagination in Weather Magic. Just in case your positive imagination is a little rusty, I'm going to give you some examples.

Let's say there was a country that was ravaged by fire. In 2019, that was the case with Australia. Someone in my online community had asked for prayers and healing for Australia, and this was going on virally throughout the internet. Having friends in Australia, I definitely had a vested interest in helping them. From experience, I've learned that Weather Magic works even better if you have a vested interest in the outcome, maybe due to the importance of emotions fueling the manifestation process.

However, as we increase our power, attention, and focus, I think we'll be equally as effective no matter whether we have a personal connection to that location or not.

I envisioned a gigantic Australian-continent-sized vacuum, sucking up the flames into a giant vacuum cleaner. Now, of course we wanted to make sure that everyone still had oxygen, so we were vacuuming only the flames in that scenario. And then, since it was raining like cats and dogs in Jakarta, according to one of my students, we decided that, hey, why not imagine all that rain getting dumped on Australia?

Within a day or two of performing weather magic, Australia ended up with a whole lot of rain, and it stopped raining in Jakarta for three days. That's an example of how you can deal with fires.

Now I'll give you another example. A friend of mine was experiencing fires in San Diego years ago, and her home was at risk of going up in flames, so she was ready to evacuate. She called out to her email list of friends for help, and she sent pictures, terrible pictures, of all sorts of devastation. I noticed that on her social media profile, she was embroiled in media drama, reliving the devastation day in and day out.

Now there's nothing wrong with being upset or anxious or fearful, especially if you're in the line of fire, literally. However, I knew that focusing on devastation wasn't doing her any good and was creating more energy toward "devastation."

Because of that, when she reached out to me and asked, "Can you do something to help the fire so I don't have to evacuate?" I instructed her I would do whatever I could to help energetically but she would have to stop focusing on the negative news and start focusing on whatever positive news she could find.

She agreed. She immediately refrained from emailing all her friends and posting terrifying photos of fires on the internet. I asked her what needed to be done to heal the fires.

She said, "We need to stop the Santa Ana winds so the firefighters can do their job."

I said, "I've got it. Thanks!"

This is what came to mind when I began Weather Magic to help her situation: I saw San Diego in my mind's eye, kind of like I was floating above a map of the area, and I saw a team of angels lined up on the coast, creating an invisible glass wall blocking the winds from coming in and blowing the fires around. The next day, my friend emailed me excitedly:

> *It's working! It's working. Whatever you're doing, it's working! The winds died down and now the firefighting planes can drop their water!*

She never had to evacuate. We both thanked the angels profusely!

There's a really important point I want to make regarding this story with my friend. Notice how important it is for us to focus our attention on what we desire, rather than what we're afraid of. This is because the energy of emotion fuels the manifestation process. If there's some weather problem somewhere in the world that you're trying to assist with, the best thing you can do is to stay off the news and stay out of the drama, with the exception of sometimes looking at an initial picture of the current circumstance in order for you to reverse or change the direction of it. But other than that, you need to stay away from the news drama and see only what you want in your mind.

And if you do happen to read a news article for facts, I want you to be very wary of the inflammatory words the media use to pull on your emotions. You know, they are selling things. That's why they use those words. The news is there to sell products and services. They have an obligation to their advertisers to sell their products, and the best way to do that is to manipulate your emotions. When you read or hear words like *devastation, pummel, wreak havoc, destruction, slam, decimate, hammer,* and *annihilate,* see if you can neutralize the resultant emotions with STOIM. Instead of getting sucked in emotionally, see if you can remain calm and neutral.

If you get all riled up, anxious, and afraid (frozen in fear), then the media have done their job. The powers that be know that when you don't access your creative potential, or Zero Point, because you are distracted by fear, they can easily manipulate you. Manipulate to do what? To buy things you don't need, to pass into law things that are potentially dangerous and inadequately tested, such as emergency vaccines. But if you know what to look out for and continue your commitment to create your own reality through Stillness, you will help bring more peace to the world.

I was once criticized in an email for not being compassionate to the plight of the Hawaiian people in the path of a hurricane, because I had warned people not to fall for the media hype. On the same day, a member of my online community thanked me for sharing my views about the hype. She lives in Hawaii. She said that when she was a child, hurricanes were normal, and she quite enjoyed seeing stuff flying around. But after she got married to a man from the mainland, any terrifying news about hurricanes would set him into a panic and her as well. After she read what I had written, she realized how calm she had been as a child and how she had become entrained to the fear of the people around her. She committed from that day forward to stop ingesting and feeding into the media hype and instead focus on what she desired: peace.

The more you can be in Stillness and see in Stillness what you desire to create—in this case, the weather you intend to create—and embody that reality as if it's already happening, despite all the people, all the news that tells you otherwise, the more powerful a person and powerful a manifester you become.

The major challenge with doing weather magic is resisting entrainment into mass consciousness or what everybody else is thinking or feeling. You will be challenged. As a last example, I'll share that, one Christmas, my husband and I were visiting his family in Texas. We were driving with his then tween-age niece back to their home. All the adults in the family were making a point to let us know how bad the weather was going to be over Christmas, how there were going to be tornadoes in that part of Texas, and how it was going to be awful.

That was the weather report on the news. While sitting in the car on the way there I turned to the niece and said, "Do you want to do some Weather Magic to change the weather so we'll have a nice Christmas?"

She looked at me with big, bright eyes and said, "Sure, how do you do that?"

I taught her what I teach you in this chapter, and warned her that she had to stay steady in that vision and feeling of the Christmas she desired, rather than get influenced by all the other adults around her who I guaranteed were going to keep talking about how bad the weather was going to be. I warned her they were going to turn on the news, and she was going to hear negative things about the weather. I warned her the other adults were not going to have the faith that Christmas was going to be beautiful. I asked her, "Can you hold your vision despite all of that challenge?"

And she said yes.

I was a proud auntie in that moment.

Over the next couple days, before Christmas came to be, every time the news came on about the weather or one of the adults lamented how bad Christmas was going to be, we gave each other knowing looks or elbowed each other, just to remind us that we were doing Weather Magic and they were not going to negatively influence us. When Christmas came, not only were there absolutely no tornadoes to be seen anywhere in the area, it was a beautiful, partly sunny day. My husband got to jump on the outdoor trampoline with his niece for hours of fun.

One of the adults in the family just happened to mention we were going to barbecue steaks and that it was too windy to barbecue. Within earshot of my niece, I just looked up at the sky, as if I was talking to God or an angel, and I said, "Hey, could you please get rid of the wind here so we can barbecue? That would be really great. Thank you so much!" Then I experienced it in my mind exactly what it would feel like to have perfect weather for barbecuing. And sure enough, the wind died down very soon afterward and we had a beautiful Christmas and a beautiful barbecue.

Chapter Summary

1. Weather Magic proves to you exactly how powerful you are.

2. Remember to use your imagination. In Stillness, you'll notice that you'll see things in your mind that will give you great ideas.

3. Remember that you can't change the weather unless it's for the highest good. At times, a storm may have to blow over on its own without any influence from us.

4. There will be challenges when you do Weather Magic because other people won't believe that it can be done. You need to have some support and a way to ignore those signals and to keep aligned with what you're creating.

Chapter 14

Travel Magic and Traffic Magic

HAPPY TRAILS. HAPPY TRIPS.

Learning Travel Magic and Traffic Magic can make your life more enjoyable on a practical level. This is very similar to Weather Magic. You apply the same skills to when you're traveling and if you have problems in traffic.

I'm sure that if you're an adult, you have experienced driving on a road in less than perfect conditions. I can cite many occasions when I was white-knuckling it through a snowstorm, anxious and fearful that, somehow, I would drive off the road and kill myself. That was before 1995, when I did slide off the road during a sudden April snowstorm and collided headlong with a tree. I was knocked out because my head hit the windshield after ricocheting back from the force of the airbag. Luckily, an off-duty EMT passed by the wreck and woke me up, rescuing me from what would have been severe burns from my engine catching fire.

There have also been times when I've been stuck in traffic for hours with no recourse, wishing that whatever accident was up ahead would clear quickly so I could get on my way. Back then I didn't know about Traffic Magic and Travel Magic.

In Traffic and Travel magic, you use the Superpowers residing in your creative potential. You get to use your powerful mind to create the image of what your future reality looks and feels like and then resonate that new reality into manifestation.

TRAFFIC MAGIC

First, let's go through the three-step process of how to do traffic magic.

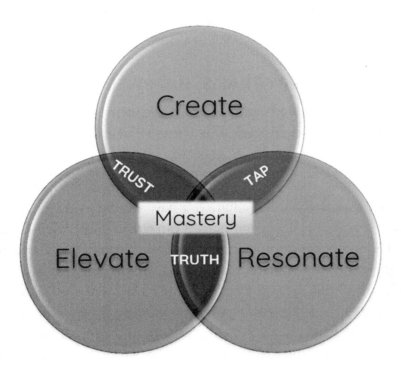

You will remember this model from when we discussed Weather Magic.

Step 1: Go into Stillness and create an image in your mind of perfect traffic. You can do this even when you are stuck in congested traffic. *Create* an image in your mind of clear roads. Whether or not you believe that the roads will clear in the near future, it's important for you to see it in your mind first. If you can, superimpose a before picture and an after picture of the traffic. Currently you're experiencing congested traffic in your reality, so you want to see the same stretch of road flowing perfectly, with ease. When you go into Stillness through STOIM, you are able to immediately access inner calm and peace. From this space, future creation is fortified. That's why we create from this space.

Step 2: *Resonate.* Using your past experiences or imagination as a template, feel that new reality already happening to you right now. In doing so, you resonate the feeling of being in flow and ease, the feeling of you driving in the car at the speed you want it to go. Resonating means feeling it in your body, not just seeing it in your mind. Most people describe that feeling as emotionally calm, peaceful, or joyful. I often feel celebratory. I usually get quite excited, celebrating my manifestation before it manifests. Maybe you will too.

Step 3: *Elevate* your emotions, purposefully tapping in to your memories or imagination of what it feels like to be emotionally calm, relaxed, and happy while traveling. You might think: *I've never felt calm, relaxed, and happy while traveling, so how am I supposed to bring up that memory?* You can tap past memories of joy and peace and apply them creatively to traveling so you can feel well.

Here's the thing: if you're always anxious driving a car and worried about bad weather or cars cutting in front of you, guess what? The Universe will comply with your intentions. Emotions are powerful attractors and your fear is like a magnet, bringing more situations that make you fearful. The Universe will then bring exactly those things you do not want tumbling into your reality. Instead, you're going to train yourself to consciously *create* your new reality, *resonate* that in your body, and consciously *elevate* positive emotions.

Masterful manifesting in our human lives is kind of like a balancing act. Imagine the old-fashioned balances they used as scales. On one side, the balance plate has fear and on the other side, the balance plate has calm, joy, or peace. The bigger the energy, the heavier the weight on either side. If your fear is a bigger energy than your joy, then the Universe has no choice but to manifest more things for you to fear.

If you have more positive emotions, they will weigh in favor of the positive image you've created. Elevating your emotions is the best way to make a big difference. If I'm in an emotional funk for whatever reason, I turn to my tools to resonate a different emotional frequency. Aside from doing TOLPAKAN Healing on myself, I've found that turning on my favorite tunes, singing out loud, or dancing around are great ways to up-level my emotions quickly.

The good news is you do not have to feel joy or bliss all the time to manifest amazing things. I've discovered the calm and peace found in STOIM is enough to manifest wondrous results without even using your creative imagination. Do STOIM as often as you can throughout the day.

One time when my husband and I were returning from a trip to Canada, we stopped by a popular doughnut shop called Tim Horton's. At the time I was hungry, so we bought some doughnut holes, called *Tim Bits*, and I decided to eat a few while driving back home. As the sugar rush and resulting sugar crash hit me soon afterward, I fell asleep while my husband continued driving. Traffic ground to a halt while I was sleeping. It was stopped cold. We could have left our car and walked around; it was that congested! At that time, I felt as if I was drugged and I wanted to continue sleeping. I could barely peel my eyes open. Then it dawned on me that the traffic was only mirroring my energy, and I knew I was being guided to do something about the situation.

Forcing myself to stay awake, I decided to do some energy work on myself and the traffic to see what would happen. As soon as my energy began returning to normal, the flow of traffic returned to normal, seemingly out of the blue. We never really did find out what the cause of the delay was.

TRAVEL MAGIC

In performing Travel Magic, you use the same three steps, but in this case, we're not just talking about traffic when you're in a car, we're talking about influencing your entire travel experience. For example, the quality of your comfort in the airplane. Say you're traveling a long distance. Ideally, you do Travel Magic days prior to leaving your home.

Step 1: To prepare, do Weather Magic for your trip. For Travel Magic, get into your BEING state through STOIM. From there, *create* in your mind what traveling in your ideal world looks like, feels like, and is like when you are there. In other words, not only are you going to prepare for smooth driving to the airport, you're going to imagine short airport lines, happy TSA agents, and happy crew members.

I usually like to do a clearing on the airport as well, so I'll actually do some TOLPAKAN healing to clear negative energy and entities from the space before I get there.

Imagine how you feel—calm and comfortable—while traveling. In the airport, for example, see yourself getting from one connection to the next with ease. See all your luggage arriving safely and securely to your final destination. Imagine feeling energized and awake when you get there. Imagine how much fun you have on the plane, watching movies or having a nice conversation, and how awesome you feel finding the exact scrumptious food you dream of at the airport. Imagine getting to your hotel or final destination with ease and speed.

Step 2: Plan your whole day in your mind before you travel. Next, you're ready to *resonate* the feeling of it already happening, or that it's already happened.

Step 3: *Elevate* your emotions to that place of calm, peace, and relaxation. You meditate on your future reality and envision what it's going to be like. That's about it. That's how you do Travel Magic— easy-peasy, right? It's not rocket science. Conscious co-creation totally rocks, and you can do it for anything in your life. If it is for the highest and greatest good, it will then manifest for you with divine timing.

I teach my TOLPAKAN Healing Level 2 Practitioner students Travel Magic Skills, such as how to pick the right line at the border crossing, but that is beyond what I can teach in this book.

Chapter Summary

1. Traffic Magic and Travel Magic are extensions of the same three steps that you use to create a new reality that serves you.

2. Start each of these manifesting exercises in Stillness, as it is the best way to get fast results.

3. Remember that being calm, peaceful, and happy is important to be able to transform your reality.

4. Conscious co-creation using the Create, Resonate, and Elevate formula can apply to all areas of your life, so have fun!

Chapter 15

Transmutational Bubble Magic

AUTO-CLEARING NEGATIVE ENERGIES

I wasn't sure I was going to include Transmutational Bubble Magic in this book. I teach it in my live event, Light Warrior Training Camp, as well as in my TOLPAKAN Healing Level 2 Practitioner Certification Program. I wasn't going to include it because to be adept, you must be at a TOLPAKAN Healing power level of 10/10. However, I am told by Source that if you are reading this book and don't yet have a TOLPAKAN healing power of 10/10, you can attain it just by doing the exercises in this book. How cool is that? That's why I was instructed to include it.

What does a TOLPAKAN Healing Power of 10/10 mean? It means you have the power to direct energy at the highest level. Your attention is so focused as to be able to heal multiple things at one time. For example, at a level of 10/10, I can heal millions of entities in the world simultaneously. I have that degree of focused attention and Stillness.

This isn't about me being any more spiritual or gifted than you. It's really about practice. Just like anything else, to become really good at something, you must focus your attention and practice. A budding virtuoso violinist may have talent, but talent is useless if she doesn't practice. Repetition and practice increase your healing power levels to the highest degree.

Transmutational Bubble Magic is a spiritual invention whereby we place a protective healing bubble just outside a person's auric or energy field. It automatically cleans and clears negative energies entering that space—as allowed by Source, of course—and it's a great way to enact spiritual protection around a loved one when you don't have overt permission to heal them. It allows you to heal the *space* around them.

There are other ways in which you can command that a Transmutational Bubble be placed around a person. You can learn to use one of my ascension healing tools, called Ascension 2 All-in-One Healing and Integration. Ascension 2 is an energy healing tool that has multiple positive morphic fields and instructions infused within it. Because this tool is doing the work for you, all you need to do is tell it *where* to place the bubble. In other words, you can use Ascension 2 and say, "Place a Transmutational Bubble around my granddaughter, please," and it will happen. The Ascension 2 tool is part of my Light Warrior Bootcamp 2.0 program as well as these positive energies being infused into my Ascension 3 Jewelry line. Refer to the Next Steps chapter for links.

If you self-muscle test that you're currently not a TOLPAKAN Healing power level of 10 and can't perform Transmutational Bubble Magic today, it doesn't mean you won't be able to in the future.

Why would you want to put a Transmutational Bubble around someone in the first place?

There are two main reasons. Reason number one: you wish to protect a friend or loved one. Reason number two: you wish to cordon off a negative influence from affecting you or others.

Imagine that around each human being, there is an auric field—an invisible field of energy outside their physical bodies that influences them and is part of who they are. Using electromagnetic devices, we can measure a field emanating from the heart, which extends like a torus—a vortex of energy—around us. The auric field is sort of like that but it is more than an electromagnetic field. It also has various mental, emotional, energetic, spiritual, and dimensional qualities to it. The health of the physical body is influenced by the health of the aura. Various books, many stemming from ancient teachings, have more information about the aura if you wish to study it. One of first set of books I read when studying as a Reiki practitioner is written by Barbara Brennen. In the books, *Light Emerging and Hands of Light*, Brennen's detailed drawings depict what the aura looks like when it is healthy and when it is not, and how our auras can interact and influence others.

Often as we go about our day, there may be people we interact with who are extremely negative; some people would even say toxic. Some are labeled *energy vampires*, because they have the amazing ability to siphon off healthy energy from others to feed themselves. I know this may sound scary if this is the first time you're hearing about it, but it doesn't have to be. By practicing Stillness through STOIM, you become increasingly sovereign, and in doing so, you prevent any sort of energy vampirism. Furthermore, with your Superpowers on lock, especially after you've discovered the Nirvana of No (see Chapter 17), you'll thwart any would-be energy vampire quickly and easily.

Here's the problem. If you have to be around an extremely negative or emotionally toxic person every day because you either live or work with them, it can be draining, no matter how good your STOIM is. This type of person is unlikely going to be open to receiving energy healing, and you may not have permission to do any healing on their behalf. If you're not allowed to heal a person because you don't have their overt permission or it's not for the highest and greatest good, then placing a Transmutational Bubble around them can be protective for you and others by keeping the negativity contained.

The other cool thing about the Transmutational Bubble is that, even if the negative person is attracting more negativity in the form of entities into their space, the minute those entities hit the boundaries of the bubble, they can be instantly healed—meaning their vibration is raised to a non-harmful level, and they can ascend to the next stage of their spiritual development. According to my conversations with Source, the Transmutational Bubble is invisible to entities, so if they enter into its space, they are automatically healed. Because entities with malevolent intent interfere with humanity's free will, we are allowed to heal them without asking permission. It's one of the exceptions to the permission rule. On rare occasion, if the human is required to deal with an entity because of the human's own soul evolution or journey, the bubble will not be allowed to automatically heal that entity.

The Transmutational Bubble contains a clearing vortex of high vibrational healing energies that sits outside a person's auric field. Because we don't have permission to download a clearing vortex *inside* of another person's auric field in many cases, this Transmutational Bubble clears the space *outside* their auric field.

I know this sounds like a back door or loophole. Well, it is. If it is for the highest and greatest good for all involved, then a Transmutational Bubble will be erected as commanded by you or your Ascension tools. Placing a Transmutational Bubble around a potentially harmful person will help protect others who might be energetically hurt by them. I would say that more than 99 percent of the time, we are allowed to create such a bubble around another person who is toxic, negative, or downright harmful to others. When we direct the download of this Transmutational Bubble, it goes outside their energy field and, like a vortex, automatically cleans and clears negative low-vibrational energy to the extent it is allowed. This includes negative energy, such as negative emotions, negative thought forms, negative entities, energy weapons, energy suckers, and the like. It also prevents entities and their weapons from escaping and harming others. As soon as they hit that bubble from the inside or from the outside, they are healed. Period.

Because you're not healing the person, you're only healing the space around them, whatever negative energy wishing to enter or exit that person will be cleared by this Transmutational Bubble. That's the idea. I created the blueprint for the Transmutational Bubble using TOLPAKAN Healing because I saw a need for it.

When might you not be allowed to download this bubble? In cases where your intended target has to deal with their own negativity or has a soul contract in place precluding the healing of an entity. But as I said before, 99 percent of the time, we're allowed to do it.

> *Please note—and this is important—that placing a Transmutational Bubble around a dangerous and abusive individual without getting outside real-world help is not appropriate. In this training, I am in no way suggesting that downloading this protective bubble is the only thing you should do. If you or a child are in danger of being harmed, you must seek the help of the authorities and get to safety as quickly as possible!*

Another instance in which you'd likely wish to perform Transmutational Bubble Magic is to protect loved ones. In that case, the space around them is constantly clearing, so wherever they may travel, it protects them. I have many clients and students with highly sensitive grandchildren who suffer when they go to school because they feel too much and come home with their auric fields dirty from the energies they've encountered during the day. Instead of begging the parents to accept energy healing or Superpower training for their children, it is sometimes more appropriate to just place a Transmutational Bubble around each one to auto-clear negative energies around them. And what I have observed is that when you do this for a loved one and whenever you think of them while in STOIM, the Transmutational Bubble you placed around them becomes bigger and stronger.

Transmutational Bubble Magic is done in three steps. They are the same three steps that we use to do Weather Magic, Traffic Magic, and Travel Magic.

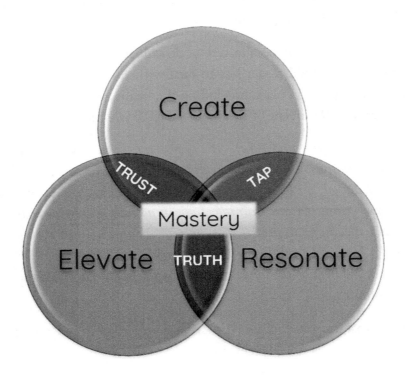

1. *Create* the bubble in your mind.

2. *Resonate* by experiencing the bubble being downloaded and activated onto the target.

3. *Elevate* your emotions by being grateful and joyful that this bubble is working.

Step 1: *Create* this bubble in your mind, what it looks like. Let's take this step by step. First, get into the BEING state, going into Stillness through STOIM. Next, create in your mind what it looks like to have a big, active cleansing bubble with a clearing vortex within it. We're talking about a bubble that surrounds the person's aura and has swirling, cleansing energies within it. Your Transmutational Bubble might look a bit different from mine, given our different imaginations. In your mind's eye, you might visualize soapsuds or scrubbers instead of a vortex. My Transmutational Bubble looks like vortices of clearing white light. Honestly, it doesn't matter if our images are different, as long as we intend what is for the highest good. I think it's whatever feels good to you. You can create it the way you want, because the intention is going to be that the energy cleans anything and everything in that space that is not 100 percent Divine Light, as allowed by Source.

Step 2: *Resonate* the feeling of clearing and cleaning the space around the person that you're targeting. This could be for yourself, your children, or your spouse. Imagine it downloading and activating onto the target person of your choice.

Step 3: *Elevate* your own emotions to get to that place of calm, relaxed, happy feeling while this is happening. That really amplifies the effect.

When I've measured the diameter of clients' or students' Transmutational Bubbles, I notice the bubble is permanent. If they go into Stillness, the bubble expands to a much larger radius compared to when they are in their waking consciousness or in a negative space. If they're in a negative space the Transmutational Bubble is still there, but it is not as wide. However, as soon as they go into STOIM or I go into STOIM while I am thinking of them, that bubble expands rapidly. Wouldn't it be great to have a really big Transmutational Bubble as you walk into a stadium full of alcohol-imbibing football fans?

In *Visions of Glory*, the author, John Pontius, describes experiencing several near-death episodes in which he could clairvoyantly see angels as well as ghosts and demons. During one of these episodes, an angel transported his spiritual body to witness spiritual activity at several places, including a bar and stadium full of fans. John was able to see ghosts and entities active in those public areas. Ghosts like to attach to living people with addictions, and demons like to attach to both ghosts and living people who resonate at a low vibrational frequency. Whether you believe in demons or ghosts is unimportant; however, it's a great overall wellness strategy to be in Stillness wherever you go, especially if you desire the Transmutational Bubble to be as large as possible.

At this point, you might be asking: "Is there a limit to how many people I can download the Transmutational Bubble for?" And the answer is, no, not that I'm aware of. You might also be wondering if you can download this Bubble to homes or objects besides living humans. The answer to that question is no. It isn't because you're not allowed, it is because you generally don't need permission to clear a space. You can directly clear the home and property internally with a clearing vortex as taught in the Light Warrior Bootcamp 2.0, rather than a Transmutational Bubble. Transmutational Bubbles are designed for living, embodied beings.

Below is the TOLPAKAN Healing Transmutational Bubble Directive. Say this while you are Creating, Resonating, and Elevating. In the blank, put in the person's name you wish to target.

> *I now command that the Transmutational Bubble be downloaded and activated to _____ in the highest and best way, in all timelines where they exist, with ease and grace. Thank you.*

That's it. Simple, right?

And here's the cool thing: We Sensitive Souls can sometimes feel what's going on in our alternate timelines. This can be problematic. So why not direct the download of the Transmutational Bubble to all your past, present, future, alternate lives simultaneously? It's up to you.

That being said, you can do one better than the Transmutational Bubble. You can clear *inside* your own auric field for all your timelines if you know how to do it and when to do it as you learned in Chapter 7 SOS Clearing. Healing multiple timelines simultaneously is a skill taught in the TOLPAKAN Healing Method Level 1 Training Program and other self-healing programs I've created.

Chapter Summary

1. Transmutational Bubble Magic can come in handy if there's someone in your life who is extremely negative.

2. Transmutational Bubble Magic requires a TOLPAKAN Healing Power Level of 10/10 to work.

3. You can check with Divine Muscle Testing what your TKH power levels are at any time.

4. Your own Transmutational Bubble expands whenever you're in Stillness, thereby increasing the healing radius.

5. Even if you don't have the power levels to create and download the Transmutational Bubble right now, you can use other tools, such as Ascension 2 (from the Light Warrior Bootcamp 2.0 Program) or Ascension 3 jewelry, to do it for you.

6. Just by regularly practicing STOIM and the other exercises in this book, you will soon reach a TOLPAKAN Power Level of 10/10.

Chapter 16

Cloud Sculpting

TELEKINESIS FOR BEGINNERS

Dr. Robert G. Jahn, a head researcher at Princeton University, did thousands of experiments on hundreds of men and women of all ages and professions and revealed that human subjects were able to move a pendulum placed under a transparent cap. They created the movement with only thought and intention in their minds. Five of those subjects were able to do it at any time and distance.[20] Other scientists have found that the power of mind can affect a variety of devices and liquid media, such as highly precise lasers, chronometers, and electrical devices.

What has telekinesis got to do with cloud sculpting?

Few people know they already possess the telekinesis blueprint. Clouds, because they are made of water vapor, are fairly easy to move with our minds. That's why I use them when teaching telekinesis. Granted, whether water vapor is indeed easier to move than, say, a pencil or a truck, is debatable because according to some theorists, it is our belief systems that block us from manifesting our true abilities.

That being said, when I've asked Source why these powers are not manifesting for everyone on the planet right now, the answer is fairly simple. It has to do with our level of consciousness. In other words, I

20 Jahn, R. G. and B. J. Dunne. "On the Quantum Mechanics of Consciousness with Application to Anomalous Phenomena." *Foundations of Physics.* 1986. 16 (8): 721–772. doi:10.1007/bf00735378

think God, the Universe, doesn't allow most of us to manifest maximum Superpowers because we haven't disciplined our minds enough to avoid inflicting harm on others. Until our mass level of consciousness resonates predominantly in the frequency of love, only certain people will be allowed to maximize their telekinetic Superpowers.

As you may have observed from stories related to heroes and villains with telekinetic powers, you could do a lot damage if you were powerfully telekinetic but lacked the discipline of controlling your emotions. What if your main motivation were to enact revenge rather than seek peace and harmony at all times?

Although I'm a fan of harnessing all Superpowers, I think we'll see an advancement of Superpowers, such as telekinesis, once we have become increasingly more conscious and able to manage our emotions, judgments, and opinions more consistently.

Cloud sculpting begins with finding a dense cloud in the sky and creating a hole in it. Yeah, it's that simple. As I said, this is the simplest way to teach Level 1 telekinesis. It's one that people can do fairly easily without their ego getting in the way.

One of the first times I taught this in a group, we had a perfect day for it—which, by the way, we created through Weather Magic. We had asked for a day with enough clouds that students could practice. If you're practicing this in a group, it's a good idea to leave each person lying down on the grass plenty of room, but I hadn't yet realized that. I had forgotten to mention that people should not work on the same cloud. Not only were some of them poking holes in the same clouds, they were getting creative, sculpting the clouds into all sorts of shapes (doughnuts, birds, dinosaurs); the clouds were bending to the will of one person, then another. We figured out that there was competition going on for the same cloud space! Well, lesson learned: it's a good idea to spread out and work on the cloud that is just above you so you're not interfering with anybody else's telekinetic intentions. Make sense?

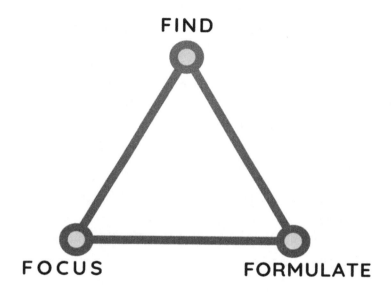

Go into a BEING state by doing STOIM before and during your cloud sculpting. You'll consume less energy this way, and you may get faster results.

In cloud sculpting, there are three steps:

1. *Find* an area of semi-dense cloud you'd like to sculpt.

2. *Formulate* in your mind's eye what it will look like after you've created a hole in it.

3. *Focus* your mind and energies in the area of cloud that you wish to sculpt.

Step 1: *Find* a dense part of a cloud that you wish to poke a hole in. Pretty easy, right? Once you've found this dense part, go ahead and lie down because it's a lot easier to do this while you're not straining your neck looking up at the sky. Lie down on a blanket or yoga mat and get comfy; look up at the cloud you'll be working on.

Step 2: *Formulate* in your mind what it will look like after you put a hole in it. Imagine the dense cloud you see right in front of you with a hole in it, okay?

Step 3: *Focus* intently, but in a relaxed way, on the density as if you were boring a hole in it or dissolving a hole in it with laser-sharp eyes. You can imagine the water vapors dissolving away in the center. Of course, you can do this in your mind's eye as well without opening your eyes if you desire. Either way is fine.

I used to think that cloud sculpting took more practice than Weather Magic because we're expecting immediate results, as compared with results that take hours or days to manifest. But I've found this just isn't true any longer. During a live event training described above, as I held the space, believing that all students would be successful, I was utterly amazed by the rapidity of the results.

When you're by yourself, be open and relaxed. If the cloud doesn't shift immediately for you, try to remain in a nonjudgmental and accepting space.

When I led this workshop at the Omega Institute in Rhinebeck, New York, we had to manifest clouds for our Cloud Sculpting class, since we had successfully manifested cloudless days using Weather Magic the week prior to the event. I requested clouds after I woke up that morning, and by the time we were ready to do the exercise, we had a giant thick blanket of cloud cover over a huge open area outside. Everyone lay on their backs, spread out on the lawn, looking at the sky.

While the students were practicing, I took the opportunity to connect with my online community via live video to share what fun we were having. I finished after a few minutes, and one of the students called me over. She looked like she was about to cry. Now I was focused on her, not looking at the sky. When I came closer to her, I could see she wasn't upset; she was in sheer disbelief.

She pointed up at the sky, and she said, "Did I really do that?"

I looked above her, and the sky was completely clear. She hadn't poked a hole in a cloud. She had decimated a baseball-field-sized cloud in a manner of minutes. And then I looked at the sky above everyone else. There wasn't a cloud left above where we were situated. Gone. The clouds were completely gone. All we could see was blue sky. It was amazing. I had allotted fifteen to twenty minutes to do this exercise, and we were done in about five.

When you're in the BEING state, and you place your intentions to *find, formulate,* and *focus* on cloud sculpting, results can appear pretty fast. As more people practice harnessing their Superpower gifts, I believe that positive manifestations will occur faster and faster worldwide. We can tap in to positive morphic fields of *already having done it.* When you harness your Superpowers, you help others connect with their abilities as well.

Cloud Sculpting is a great introduction to telekinesis. If you want more advanced telekinesis training, I highly suggest that you watch the film *Superhuman* by Caroline Cory and participate in a workshop to learn more advanced skills.

Please teach this to your young children or grandchildren. It is fun to do, and it proves to them that they have immense power when they can connect to their BEING state and focus on a positive intention. You might find they have some really creative ways of changing the clouds. Please feel free to share your results in my private online community.

Chapter Summary

1. Telekinesis is a skill and gift that many of us aspire to. Many of us do not practice because we don't believe we can do it.

2. Cloud sculpting is a simple, elegant, and quick way of performing beginner telekinesis without worrying about harming another person or getting drained by trying too hard.

3. Our abilities to perform telekinesis on a bigger scale, such as moving a truck with our minds, may be currently regulated by our level of consciousness as a human collective.

4. Cloud sculpting is a fun way to show children how powerful they are, so please teach it to your children and grandchildren, and have fun.

Chapter 17

Nirvana of No

WHY SAYING NO SUPPORTS YOUR SUPERPOWERS

Are you too nice?

Do you get kudos for being *nice, helpful, the rock, the problem-solver, the angel,* or *always there for people?*

I find it fascinating to hear what extraordinarily successful people share about the importance of being able to say no. In a Forbes business article,[21] Steve Jobs was quoted as saying, "Focusing is about saying no." Warren Buffett said, "We need to learn the slow yes and the quick no." And Tony Blair, former prime minister of Britain, said, "The art of leadership is saying no, not saying yes. It is very easy to say yes."

What does saying no have to do with our Superpowers?

When we are true to ourselves, we bring all of our power back. When we have all of our power back and all of our circuits fully charged, we can harness and express amazing abilities. That includes intuiting, healing, creating, and manifesting abilities.

When we aren't able to say no to people because of guilt, shame, fear, or codependency, we deposit energetic parts of ourselves elsewhere and are no longer cohesive, fully realized humans. To fully harness

---

21 Becher, Jonathan. "Six Quotes to Help You Understand Why It's Important to Say No." *Forbes.* Aug 12, 2015. forbes.com/sites/sap/2015/08/12/quotes-on-saying-no/#7334026b5555

your sensitivity as a Superpower, you need to develop the ability to say no. Then, you need to practice saying no. That's why this chapter is just as important as all the other ones in this book.

I want you to imagine I'm throwing a ball and you're going to catch it. What would happen if I threw you just one ball? You probably would have a pretty good chance of catching it. But what if I threw three, four, or five balls at you in rapid succession? Would you be able to catch them all? Chances are that you're going to drop some, right? And even if you are a good juggler, there's a limit to how many balls you can juggle in the air at one time. Not being able to say no is like that: you are juggling multiple balls and not doing a very good job.

Not saying no is *exhausting*. If you are already tired and exhausted, look to your ability or inability to say no in situations and circumstances that don't serve you.

I know, I know. We've grown up with the notion that serving ourselves is *selfish*, but I've come to the stark realization that if our only responsibility were to serve others, then other people have the responsibility to serve us. When we expect others to serve us, we don't always get what we want, nor what we deserve, because we are putting the responsibility to serve us squarely in their hands. Who knows us better than we do? Nobody. When we all serve everyone to the exclusion of ourselves, nobody is happy.

You may already be arguing: *But Dr. Karen, I can't say no to my husband!* or *Dr. Karen. I can't say no to my children!* or *Dr. Karen, I can't say No to my boss, can I?*

The answer is yes; yes, you can! Say no when it's appropriate for two reasons:

1. Only you truly know and appreciate your own limits.

2. The Universe will mirror to you how you're treating yourself.

If you consistently disrespect and ignore your wants and needs, the Universe will bring more people who will do the same to you.

Kind of sucks, doesn't it?

Let me say it another way: If you allow yourself to be continually drained, put upon, or depended on, then the Universe will continue presenting to you the similar energies and situations that cause you to be drained, put upon, and depended on. Stop being a martyr. It's a cop out—and now you know it. Martyring ourselves is an underhanded way we shirk our personal responsibilities to be at the helm of our lives, giving us the opportunity to blame others for our situations and how we feel.

You can either be victimized or empowered. You can't be both simultaneously. You choose.

If you want freedom from the kind of codependent life that makes it other people's fault that you are suffering, then you need to have the courage to step up, say no, and have the faith that doing what is best for you is what is best for all involved (even if you can't see it right away). Have faith that the Universe will help the other person in a way that doesn't involve you. If you habitually go into rescue mode, it blocks others from stepping into their power. You're half the problem! So, stop it already.

Am I being harsh, or am I being honest?

I sometimes joke about my former self being a poster child for codependency, meaning that I was absolutely horrible at saying no. I would say yes all the time because I felt bad that I wanted to help every single person on the planet, not realizing I was harming both myself and my relationships in the process.

Decades ago, I was in the back room of a medical clinic with a patient when, suddenly, I heard loud wailing noises coming from the front office. At first, I thought it was somebody being rowdy, and I was just about to peek out the door to hush whoever it was. But then I realized the sound was someone crying. After composing myself, I finished with my patient and went to the front desk to ask my staff what was going on. Apparently, the receptionist's husband had just died in a car accident, and the state trooper had come by to let her know. She was the one wailing.

I felt terrible for her. But as days and weeks went by, I felt even worse for her, and the reason was this: Her late husband was someone who said yes to everybody. He was a sweet, generous soul. Unfortunately, because he said yes to everybody, he gave whatever he had to those in need and left his wife and two children with no savings, no insurance, and no protection.

He was so busy helping other people he didn't realize the potential harm he was doing to his family. He would have lent the shirt off his back if it helped somebody else. Everyone in town loved him. But his family suffered for it, and he had no idea he was doing that to them because, of course, he had no idea he was going to die as a young man.

By saying yes to everyone else, you may be saying no to yourself, your dreams, and your loved ones.

Learning to say no is also instructing the Universe in how you like to be treated. I said it before, but I'll say it again in a different way: How you treat yourself will be mirrored in your future reality. Whatever you're saying yes to, the Universe says, "Okay, I'll give you more of that." If you're saying yes to people and situations that don't resonate with you because you're feeling obliged to, then the Universe will give you more of that.

Yucky, if you ask me. Been there. Done that. I had to get physically sick to the point of being disabled before I learned to say no. I hope you don't need as much motivation as I did.

Another reason we highly Sensitive Souls in particular say yes when we want to say no is that Sensitive Souls get a double dose. In other words, not only do we get the negative energy coming toward us if someone reacts negatively to us when we say no, we also get to feel *their* negative energy in *our* bodies because we are naturally empathic. We are afraid of the other person's reaction. We can feel empathically the other person's sadness, anger, or disappointment in their bodies as if it were our own. We get a double whammy, which definitely does not feel good. To avoid this discomfort, we say yes even when we want to say no.

I get it. Being sensitive can suck if you're constantly feeling other people's negative emotions. It can be draining and overwhelming. I've been there too. Instead of allowing the other person to have a reaction, we try to control the situation by avoiding the reaction. But we do this at a cost. It costs us our power to create our lives.

We say yes because we don't want all that emotional and energetic baggage. That is not a good enough reason to say yes. Ultimately, *you* are responsible for the baggage you do and do not take on. It's not necessary, even if the person has a reaction, to assume their negative energy and emotions. With practice and plenty of compassion to allow the other person the space to have a reaction without trying to change or control them, you will develop the skills needed to not take on their stuff.

I remember reading Melody Beatty's *Codependent No More*, in which she chastises codependent people—people who are too nice—for being control freaks. At first when I read it, I was quite offended by this criticism. But then I realized she was spot on. My saying yes instead of no was my way of avoiding the reaction from the other person and, in essence, controlling them by not giving them a choice to have a reaction. Hence, I was being a control freak or, in other words, *I was controlling*.

Not a very attractive trait, especially for someone who prided herself in being *nice*.

Understanding that my codependency was self-serving and controlling burst my belief bubble of *I'm a nice girl*. At that pivotal moment when I became conscious of this pattern, I decided to change it.

Change was a rocky road, and to this day, I continue to heal deeper, subtler layers of residual codependency. Relinquishing control can be challenging, but at least I'm more self-compassionate when that control monster rears its ugly head.

Is saying no a challenge for you? Well, I wouldn't be surprised if you say it is. If you're not used to saying no, saying no is going to feel very awkward at the beginning and maybe even scary. I know that as a kind, sensitive person, you probably want to deliver a no as gently and nicely as possible. However, if you're not well practiced in saying no, when it finally blurts out of your mouth, it can come out a little rough. My first spiritual teacher, Pat Jones, told me that when we are too nice, it's like a pendulum that swings in only one direction. When we heal these patterns, sometimes the pendulum has to swing all the way to the opposite side for us to find the balance point.

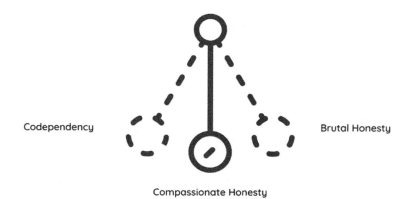

Codependency

Brutal Honesty

Compassionate Honesty

I'm giving you a heads-up that you won't be perfect at the beginning. Sometimes, years of resentment finally come pouring out when you first heal codependency patterns. It's like a bottle of soda that has been shaken, and you're finally opening the top for the first time. It simply explodes. Unless you are already prone to emotional explosions (which means you're not able to contain or transmute uncomfortable energies efficiently), it's unlikely you're going to hurt anyone with the truth.

Be patient with yourself. You might think you're screwing up at the beginning and that's okay. Is it possible you might hurt someone's feelings? Yes, it's possible. But you and I know it is not your intention, and you have to remember that each person is responsible for their own emotions. You are not responsible for their emotions, just yours.

I grow annoyed when I sense someone is being codependent with me. They are being inauthentic. Authenticity is the *new black*, meaning it is in style. Being honest and authentic are qualities that everyone appreciates.

You might find this a bit humorous, but one time after blurting out a no to someone, without first couching it gently, I said, "Whoops! That came out a little blunt. Sorry about that!"

And you know what? They might have looked a little shocked at first, but they got over it quickly. Why? Because they didn't take it personally. The best thing about being habitually honest, and I mean really honest—about how you feel and what your preferences are—is that others learn to *trust* you.

Coming up are some "no" scripts. I love scripts. Scripts are helpful because many of us don't know how to say no nicely. Having a script we can practice when we're not in the heat of the moment can help us become more confident when those situations come up. We'll also be less likely to blurt out something hurtful due to pent-up resentment.

Here are some scripts you can use when people ask you to do something and you don't want to do it.

> **"I'd love to help, but I've got to focus on what's on my plate right now."**

Pretty simple, right?

Here's another one:

> **"That's not going to work for me, and _____ (state your preferences)."**

For example: "That's not going to work for me and I truly appreciate you thinking of me." Or "That's not going to work for me and I'll have more available time in about three weeks."

Notice the use of *and* rather than *but*, and how it changes the feeling of the statement. When you use the word *and*, it is inclusive and doesn't create a stoppage of energy. It's more positive, in other words.

> **"This isn't resonating right now with me, and if something changes, I'll let you know."**

Again, you can use the word *but*. We're choosing to use the word *and* instead.

This one is great if you happen to be a person who immediately says yes because it feels good in the moment. I'm one of those people who absolutely loves saying yes. I am learning to pause longer before saying yes because, if someone is super-excited about my being involved, I get easily wrapped up in *their* excitement. Sometimes being highly sensitive can be a downfall if we're not careful. Some of the excitement and enthusiasm I feel in my body might not be mine.

If you are someone who easily jumps the gun and then regrets it later, practice this script:

"Give me some time to feel it out, and I'll get back to you."

Cool, right? Yeah, it's a good one to memorize.

Here's one that shares a little more vulnerability. If you are courageous, you may want to try this script, especially for those close to you. When you can be vulnerable in a good way with people you trust, it increases the intimacy of that relationship. And boy, does it feel good when you're able to do it. I can tell you firsthand, it's incredibly liberating to be that real, that authentic, that honest.

"I tend to say yes too quickly and end up disappointing myself and others. So, let me get back to you on this by _____ (date).

You're giving yourself some quiet time to contemplate your answer, and there is nothing wrong with that. Notice how this script is honest, authentic, and vulnerable without being self-critical. Try it out and see if you like it. Practice this with people you love and trust.

Christine Carter has written a great article with additional handy scripts, called "Five Research-Based Ways to Say No." You can find it at *Greater Good* magazine.[22]

Your home*play* (instead of home*work*) is to make up more of your own responses. Maybe you know a friend or two who could use some help saying no as well, and you can get together and have a script-writing party.

Two of the easiest and most effective scripts are:

"This isn't going to work for me."

"This isn't resonating right now."

---

22 Carter, Christine. "Five Researched-Based Ways to Say No." *Greater Good Magazine.* 25 November 2015. greatergood.berkeley.edu/article/item/5_research_based_ways_to_say_no#thank-influence

These responses do not invite any counterargument. If you create excuses, others can argue those excuses away. For example, your excuse might be, "Oh, I've got too much to do tonight. I've got to feed and walk the dog . . . and I've got to help Jimmy with his homework." The other person might pose a counterargument, "Well, why don't you ask John to feed and walk the dog and help Jimmy with his homework? It's about time he helped you out, don't you think?" Then you're left with arguing back or coming up with new excuses. Not a good scene.

What happens if someone you say no to has a negative reaction? *Allow* them the space to react, and remember you are not responsible for their emotions. You are responsible for your own. It is important that you do not take their reactions personally. In other words, it isn't your fault that they are having a negative reaction. We're human; we are all apt to react to something at some time without having conscious control. It's okay. That's where compassion comes in. Lying is not compassionate. Telling your truth is.

You can develop some scripts for these situations, too, if you like, such as:

"I'm sorry you're feeling disappointed."

"This is probably not what you wanted to hear."

"I empathize with how you might feel."

Refrain from trying to rescue them from feeling bad. Sometimes I remind myself it is my ego that thinks I'm the only one who can solve their problem. That reminds me that when one door closes, another one opens. In other words, when we're acting self-responsibly, the Universe colludes to support the best outcome for all. Often the solutions manifested are more miraculous and synchronistic than we could ever have guessed, as long as we do our part.

The Universe knows I'm pretty good at saying no most of the time when it is appropriate, and to deepen my resolve, my discernment, and my trust in the Divine, it's been giving me harder challenges lately. It's easy to say no to the random telemarketer wanting to sell something I don't need—by the way, I think this is a good example of whom to practice on first. It's also easy to say no to friends who want me to do something I know isn't going to work for me. It's even getting easier saying no to my family, which is notoriously difficult for most people. Lately, I've had to learn to say no to my energy healing colleagues and friends. That has proven to be much harder for me because I know their hearts have good intentions, and they are bringers of the Light.

Energy healers have a habit of trading sessions for each other when the time arises, and I've done my fair share. I've had to say no to many healers who have asked to offer me a healing in exchange for my testimonial if I get positive results or a reciprocal healing on them. It's a thing we do for each other; however, I can no longer spare the time or energy in this space.

Take my friend, "Libby," for example. She is a respected energy healer, and I met her through our coach. I didn't know her all that well but met her in person at an event. Because of that familiarity, I began receiving Facebook Messenger messages from her about how, in her words, her financial situation was *f*cked*, and she was in a state of utter despair. I felt bad for her. It sounded like she had asked many of her energy healing colleagues to do readings on her, and yet she was no better. As a professional courtesy, I did one mini-reading for her. I didn't even think to charge her for it because I give mini-readings and healings to my online community once a month anyway. That's what I said to myself to justify my actions.

The Universe told me in no uncertain terms, however, that although I could tune in and do a mini-reading, I was not allowed to do the healing. I shared with her my assessment and told her exactly what needed to be healed and that she had every capability to do the healing herself.

Then, I probably went a little overboard and gave her some advice. I felt it was justified, given that she was asking for my help. I told her she didn't need a bunch of free readings or healings from other healers. Instead she needed to hire one coach who could help guide her. I felt strongly she needed to invest in a coach and trust the Universe in the process. I even arranged for her to have a free twenty-minute mentoring session with a mentor who could help.

Energy healers can be cheap when it comes to investing in ourselves. Okay—that was a little rude, but I'm including myself in that description, or my former self, anyway. We are okay with investing hundreds or thousands of dollars in learning a healing modality or exploring our inner child with some big-name guru on another continent, but we are not okay with spending money on coaching when we will be *accountable* to someone who will get us to where we need to go. I'm not talking about any old coach. I'm talking about the *right* coach or mentor.

In Libby's case, although she appreciated my reading, she didn't take action on any of my other advice. Not long afterward, she wrote me again, asking me to do another reading on her. Not once did she offer to pay me or even ask if I was taking new clients. She didn't even ask me if she could reciprocate in some way valuable to me. Such was her scarcity mindset at the time. When I asked her why she didn't follow through on speaking with the mentor, she skirted the question.

Upon this second request for a free reading, I had to put my foot down. I knew I had to say no. Part of me wanted to rescue her and fix her because that's what she wanted. She respected my modality and its precision, but she was not respecting my time nor energy. I'd be lying if I said it was easy to say no. It wasn't. But, lucky for me, I had been practicing saying no, even to my friends and colleagues, for a number of years. I went into Stillness, asked for guidance on what to say, and then wrote my reply with as much love energy attached to it as I could muster.

I wrote:

> *I'm pretty sure I won't be able to help you, and I'm so sad to say this to you. I have to stop doing Band-Aid fixes for people, especially when they aren't ready to take my counsel to heart (which is perfectly okay, but just not a good fit). But know that I love you!*

Libby was very disappointed, and I could feel it on my end, so I held the space for it.

The vibe I was sending to her was unconditional love and the feeling of *You can do this! I believe in you!* I knew deeply in my heart that saying no was the best thing for her, even if none of her other energy healing friends could say no. I was relieved when she said she respected my position and she never asked me for free help again.

The best part of the story is that, several months went by, and I happened upon a beautiful picture of her launching a brand-new program. Not only that, she had co-authored a book. Seeing that shot waves of joy through my heart. She had done it! If I hadn't said no when I needed to say no, she might be in a different place. No one knows for sure, but sometimes saying no has a positive effect even if you never recognize it.

In my books, the most masterful healers aren't those who are the most clairvoyant, nor are they those who get the best tangible results. Healing is not a competition. The most masterful healers grow and challenge themselves every day, becoming ever-more conscious. That means questioning their own beliefs, habits, and judgments, doing what is hard rather than what is easy when Divinely Aligned; and being willing to receive negative feedback that bruises the ego, rather than looking for kudos that bolsters the ego.

Here's something you need to know: You do not have to explain why you are saying no. You can simply say "No, this doesn't work for me." That's it. No long explanations, no reasons, no excuses. Not wanting to do it is reason enough. Period.

Once you master the art of saying no, you'll understand why I call it the *Nirvana of No*. The amount of freed-up energy to manifest and create your life anew will be bountiful. I look forward to hearing your personal results, so feel free to share your Nirvana of No wins in my online community.

Chapter Summary

1. Being able to say no and release codependent patterns is absolutely essential for harnessing your Superpowers because by being true to yourself, you get your power back.

2. Sometimes it is easy for sensitive people to say yes because they get enmeshed in the other person's emotions instead of staying sovereign.

3. Practice with scripts when you're not with another person, so that when you are in a situation in which you want to say no, you are prepared.

4. Saying no takes courage, so be gentle with yourself for not being perfect at it right away.

5. Once you get good at saying no, you'll notice that you'll be able to say it with more ease and confidence, and it won't seem hard any longer.

6. When you are tempted to say yes but you really want to say no, remember it's most likely because you are afraid and want to be in control. Being a controlling person, however, has never made anyone happy.

7. Allow others the freedom to have a reaction, and don't take it personally.

8. Your ability to be honest and authentic will free up energy that you can use to create the life of your dreams.

Chapter 18

Superpower Mastery

TIME TO LEVEL-UP

Congratulations! By reading this book and training your Superpowers, you are evolving yourself to a new level of self-empowerment most people never dream of. I am grateful and humbled that you've taken this journey with me.

I don't know about you, but I get a lot of mileage and knowledge just by reading books. At the same time, I realize that the quantum leaps in my growth have occurred mainly when one of two things happens: I go to a live event or receive expert mentoring and coaching.

What does that mean for you? Let's talk first about live events and why they rock.

When I'm at home, I easily get distracted. I have business stuff to do, home stuff to do, and miscellaneous stuff to do. I might intend to do an online workshop training, and even block out three hours to do it, but life gets in the way. It's not that I don't do it if I really want to do it; it just takes me a heck of a lot longer than I first thought.

The same applies when I read books. The best track record I have for reading and finishing a book is being on an airplane. Yup. Without access to my Facebook Messenger or business email, I get undistracted time to read and write books (and create healing programs) on the plane.

I understand busy people don't always take the time to do all the exercises in a book. They read the book but don't do the work. While I'm highly productive, there are many times I've read a book and thought to myself: *Yeah, I'll do that exercise later*, but I never get around to it.

That's why live events rock. Without Facebook, email, phone, shopping, cooking, cleaning, and other activities of daily life distracting me, I can fully immerse myself in the learning and transformational experience during a live event. I can be fully present.

Most people benefit from a live training event with me because not only do they get valuable feedback and confirmation that they've learned the skills, but they have the opportunity to ask questions specific to their circumstances. At live events, I get to tailor the training with participant-specific energetic healing. That means that every person leaves the training knowing how to self-muscle test, change the weather, and safely practice some form of telekinesis. That also means that significant mental, emotional, energetic, or spiritual blocks preventing them from stepping into the next phase of their Superpower development are resolved on the spot. Finally, it means that they are confident that they can perform remote energy healing on another person safely and easily.

The second thing that grows me by leaps and bounds is investing in a mentor or coach who has the experience of knowing how to move me from where I am to where I want to be. I used to balk at investing in coaching because I had the erroneous belief that I could do it all on my own. Well guess what? No one who was ever happy, successful, and impacted many lives ever did it without at least one mentor or coach. Usually it is more than one. I heard one of my coaches years ago share that, even though she is a celebrity millionaire-maker coach, she has upward of eight coaches herself.

Every mentor I have worked with has helped me overcome blocks I didn't know I had and has catapulted me to the next level of personal development and success. That doesn't mean I didn't resist the help. For instance, one of my mentors, Jim, suggested I hire an office assistant for my acupuncture practice because I was coming home late every night, tired of doing menial work (like putting price labels on my supplements). I fought him on this piece of advice because I told him I couldn't afford it. He asked me how much I thought my time was worth per hour. At the time, I answered $150 per hour. He said to me, "Okay. So why are you doing a $10 an hour job?"

Back then, I didn't understand how my frustration and vibration of lack and scarcity was pushing away abundance. Finally, Jim convinced me. I called up a recently retired friend of mine, asking her if she would work as an office assistant for me. I told her I wasn't sure when I could pay her, but she was okay with that. She did it out of the goodness of her heart.

But you know what happened?

Within three weeks, my office practice became booked solid. Every appointment slot was filled! New patients were approaching me left, right, and center. Not only was I able pay her, I was making more money and no longer worried about paying the rent.

After that experience with my coach, I never doubted him—or expert coaching—again.

Being a tad stubborn and proud in the past, I had to be fed up big-time before I would ask for help. I had a million reasons why it wouldn't work. Not enough money, not enough time, the list goes on. But you know what? When I had exhausted every avenue of learning on my own, I finally took the plunge. Investing in a mentor multiplied my success by ten times. For example, in 2016, I had invested $7,000 in a coaching program. Within a year, my return on investment was over $70,000.

These days, I have no qualms about investing in mentoring and coaching. I understand the true value of getting the right help at the right time from the right person.

What if you could know exactly what needs to heal and how to heal it, quickly, easily and gracefully? What if you knew the perfect question to ask about how to resolve your symptoms today? What if you understood your Soul Mission and cleared all the blocks preventing you from stepping into your true power? What would your life look like then?

Now you might be wondering: *What else can I do with my Superpowers, now that I know I have them?*

The answer: *Lots!*

Many Sensitive Souls naturally gravitate to healing and helping professions. This is, of course, not by accident. We're natural helpers and healers. If you've held a dream of being an energy healer, or even if you are one right now, there are ways to train and practice healing at a very high level. In my TOLPAKAN Healing Method Level 1 Training Program (TKH), I teach you how to ask quality questions of the Divine to figure out what wants to heal in your life and how to heal it with frequencies of energy.

TKH complements other forms of healing, so if you are trained in another modality, you can benefit even more from learning TKH. The one thing that sets TOLPAKAN Healing apart from other methods of healing is being able to ask precise, quality questions so you can home in on what needs to heal and how.

For example, say you're suffering from knee pain, and whatever you've already done to try to alleviate it, including seeing your doctor, isn't helping. With TOLPAKAN Healing, we can ask very specific questions about your knee pain by first connecting with Source, and then performing Divine Muscle Testing.

My friend, Oliver, had such a pain. The doctor diagnosed bursitis and tried to aspirate some joint fluid, but couldn't find any. He had no other explanation for Oliver's symptoms. I demonstrated the TKH method and, within a few minutes, determined that the symptom was linked to some sort of energetic weapon from a past life. Within minutes after removing it with TOLPAKAN Healing, Oliver was able to sprint up and down the block without any pain.

TOLPAKAN healing is particularly adept at healing and releasing insidious, harmful energies that other modalities cannot. That includes spiritual imbalances that are commonly discussed in many cultures but taboo to discuss in the West: curses, energy weapons, and negative entities or spirits.

There are three TKH Healing Guides. In each guide is a table or matrix of common answers you can test for with Divine Muscle Testing to pinpoint the cause or contributing factors to a particular symptom. Then using TOLPAKAN Healing Directives, you can direct healing frequencies to support the resolution of these factors with ease and speed.

Graduates of TKH Level 1 Training can apply to join the TOLPAKAN Healing Method Level 2 Practitioner Certification Training Program to become certified in the modality and become a professional healer.

To learn more about the TOLPAKAN Healing Method or any of my self-healing programs, go to my website listed in Next Steps.

Beyond learning my healing method, there are other tools that can support you in thriving as a Sensitive Soul. My free Clearing and Protection Spray Formula (link listed in Next Steps) is an energy-infused water-charging program that can help you maintain healthier energetic spaces around you. You can use the formula to charge a spray bottle of water with energies that can clear negative energies around you or in your home. If you have highly sensitive children, it's a great idea for them to decorate their own spray bottle with light and fun stickers or bling, so that they can be motivated to clear themselves regularly.

If you find that your highly sensitive child is anxious, grumpy, or acting out, it's likely that they are feeling and sensing negative energy. As their parent, it's important that you teach them some of the skills I've taught you in this book. When these become everyday habits, your children will be able to thrive in any stressful environment.

The best way to help your children is through modeling. Parents sometimes feel like they must pretend to be okay when they are not so their children feel safe and don't have to worry about them. Unfortunately, children are naturally intuitive and can see right through the facade. If you are stressed and having a bad day, instead of pretending you're fine, why not enlist your children to support you? You can ask them to spray you with the Clearing and Protection Spray Formula so you can feel better. Not only will they have a bit of fun squirting water all over you, they'll feel good knowing they can help you. I wish I had possessed a tool like this when I was growing up because my mother was depressed, and I felt helpless. If I had known of something to help her feel better, I would've done it! By modeling that it's okay to ask for help, your children will likely ask you to spray them when they are stressed.

That is exactly what happened with a client's thirteen-year-old son. "Taylor" was having sudden, explosive bouts of violence and frustration toward his baby sister. His mother wasn't sure how best to help him and was ready to ship him off to live with his father. I recognized that Taylor was highly sensitive and he was acting out because of the negative energy he brought home from school that he couldn't effectively clear, contain, or transmute.

I first reassured Taylor there wasn't anything wrong with him. Much of his discomfort was because he was highly gifted. Then we demonstrated the clearing spray on his mom. We got Taylor to spray her, after which she smiled and thanked him. Then I asked him if he wanted to try it and he said yes. Mom got to spray him and a few seconds later, we asked him how he felt. He answered, "Calm."

Next, I asked him if he was willing to help spray his mom whenever she was feeling stressed and out of sorts. He cheerily agreed. I suggested if he ever felt like he was going to explode—because that's what it feels like for a kid overwhelmed with energies—he could always ask his mom to spray him. We all agreed that it was a plan.

A couple weeks later, I connected with the mother and asked how Taylor was. She said he was doing great. He came home one day, made a bee-line for the clearing spray bottle, and said, "Mom! Spray me, please!" Taylor had recognized that he didn't feel well and was ready to explode. He had reached out for help. Within minutes he was back to his kind, loving, sensitive self. The family was at peace, and there were no more episodes of violence against his baby sister.

I recently asked people before joining the tribe of Sensitive Souls in my private online community group to name three things that bothered them the most. One of these answers was the pain of feeling isolated and disconnected from Source, their tribe, and people who understand them. I understand this kind of pain. *You don't have to be alone.*

Now that you've connected with me in this book, let's connect you to our bigger tribe so you can thrive among people who are sensitive, just like you, and who help, support, and send positive intentions for each other. The best way to be connected is to join my private online community called Light Warrior Network (see links in Next Steps).

It's free to join. You'll need to answer a few qualifying questions just to make sure you're a good fit for the group.

The purpose of the group is to support, encourage, and inspire each other. Every month I do a free mini-reading/healing. Just get on my mailing list to find out when the next mini-reading/healing session is scheduled. Please join the Light Warrior Network group today so you can connect with the rest of our Sensitive Soul tribe.

I'm sending you my love and blessings!

Next Steps

Here are some handy links to resources I've mentioned in the book.

COMMUNITY

Join the free private online community: **LightWarriorNetwork.com**

FREEBIES

Clearing and Protection Spray™ Formula:
ClearingandProtectionSpray.com

Sensitive Soul Empowerment Guide: **SensitiveSoulGuide.com**

Stillness-on-the-Fly™ Training and MP3 download:
StillnessontheFly.com

TRAINING

Join the next Light Warrior Training Camp™ live event:
LightWarriorTrainingCamp.com

Learn more about the TOLPAKAN™ Healing Method Level 1
Training Program: **TolpakanHealingMethod.com**

TOLPAKAN™ Healing Method Level 2 Practitioner Certification
Training Program: see contact information below to find out more.

SELF-HEALING PROGRAMS

Sensitive Soul SOS™ – a foundational program for quickly decreasing
sensitivity symptoms in Sensitive Souls: **SensitiveSoulSOS.com**.

Light Warrior Bootcamp 2.0™ and Ascension 1 & 2 tools – a
program to learn how to clear entities and negative influences

from yourself, your space, your electronics and your sleep realms: **LightWarriorBootcamp.com**.

Holistic Health Transformation Program – a holistic health program that includes body-mind-spirit teachings to live a happier, healthier lifestyle: **HolisticHealthTransformationProgram.com**.

Other self-healing programs not mentioned in this book can be found on **KarenKan.com**.

ASCENSION 3 JEWELRY

I've created a line of jewelry for men, women, and children, including teethers for babies, that are energetically infused with healing energies. Each product is infused with energies of my Ascension 1 Clearing and Protection, Ascension 2 Healing and Integration, Hiddenite gem, Schumann EMF Protection, and the Flower of Life. They help Sensitive Souls stay calm, supported, and protected.

Learn more at **Ascension3.net**

PRIVATE HEALING AND MENTORING

If you're the kind of person who likes efficiency (like I do) and wants to reach your goals without struggling to try to figure it out all by yourself, or spending time learning my healing modality first, then maybe expert healing and mentoring is for you. Apply for a *Discovery Interview* to find out more about my VIP Transformational Programs, where you get to work one-on-one with me privately, and whether we are a good fit for each other. Go to **KarenKan.com/VIP** to learn more.

FINAL THOUGHTS . . .

You're not alone. There are people who understand you, what you've been going through, and the challenges you face. I want to see you thrive as a Sensitive Soul so we can all shine our light and pull the world out of darkness. We need you to be the best version of you, and it's my mission to get you there. If you need help, please reach out!

You can contact me via **KarenKan.com/CONTACT**

About the Author

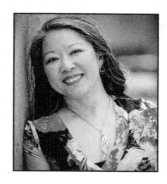

Karen Kan, MD, is a Doctor of Light Medicine, number-one bestselling author, speaker, workshop leader, energy healer, and the Founder of the Academy of Light Medicine and the TOLPAKAN Healing Method.

Dr. Karen's mission is to empower highly sensitive people to harness their Superpowers, fulfill their purpose, and create a life of joy. Through her Academy, Dr. Karen teaches the three-step TOLPAKAN Healing Method (TKH), which involves aligning with Divine Source, asking quality questions through Divine Muscle Testing, and activating specific healing frequencies.

Dr. Karen has a degree in biochemistry and medicine. She graduated magna cum laude in the top ten of her medical school class and became an assistant professor at UCLA. After graduation and almost a decade of delivering babies and treating thousands of patients in underserved communities, Dr. Karen succumbed to fibromyalgia, chronic fatigue syndrome, and autoimmune disease. Tapping in to natural healing resources, including energy and spiritual medicine, Dr. Karen was able to heal herself. She has since gone on to win multiple national and international gold medals in three disciplines of adult figure skating: singles, pairs, and ice dance.

Dr. Karen is a faculty presenter at the prestigious Omega Institute and the International Academy of Universal Self-Mastery and is a popular speaker on multiple telesummits, including "You Wealth Revolution," "From Heartache to Joy," "Elevated Existence," and "Wisdom of the Ancients." On her Light Warrior Radio podcast, she interviews the best thought leaders and healers of our time to empower others to create the life of their dreams.

56 STOIM
57 Focus/Feel/Flow
i80

57908610R00139